Stephane Cássia O. R. Vexenat
Noeme Sousa Rocha

Cytodiagnosis

Stephane Cássia O. R. Vexenat
Noeme Sousa Rocha

Cytodiagnosis

Unesp Botucatu Veterinary Hospital - Standardization, Implementation, Monitoring

ScienciaScripts

Cover image: www.ingimage.com

This book is a translation from the original published under ISBN 978-613-9-67655-2.

Publisher:
Sciencia Scripts
is a trademark of
Dodo Books Indian Ocean Ltd. and OmniScriptum S.R.L publishing group

120 High Road, East Finchley, London, N2 9ED, United Kingdom
Str. Armeneasca 28/1, office 1, Chisinau MD-2012, Republic of Moldova, Europe
Printed at: see last page
ISBN: 978-620-8-17587-0

index

Thanks

Developing a project of this size involves a huge population taking part: some with their teachings and suggestions; others with the manufacture, care, maintenance and supplies. To all those who, directly or indirectly, made this work possible, facilitating and smoothing the way, my deepest gratitude.

Special recognition is dedicated:

To the Department of Pathology of the Faculty of Medicine of UNESP Botucatu, for allowing me to circulate freely in its diagnostic routine, scientific meetings, consultations, classes, contributing to my professional improvement, as well as for having encouraged me to apply the knowledge acquired in the veterinary environment.

To the Professors, Residents and Staff of the Small and Large Animal Clinic, Veterinary Surgery and Anesthesiology, Veterinary Reproduction and Radiology and Infectious Diseases of the Veterinary Hospital of UNESP Botucatu, for their vote of confidence in the implementation of the cytological examination.

To the Veterinary Pathology Residents, who have already completed the program and those who are about to, for their tireless participation in all stages of this work.

To the postgraduates, undergraduates and interns for their attention and collaboration in this work.

To the Professors and Staff of the Veterinary Pathology department, for their friendship and support in carrying out the work.

To FUNDUNESP, for financing the first reagents and equipment for collecting and processing the cytological samples.

To FAPESP and CAPES, for the grants that made it possible to generate knowledge and train human resources in the field.

1. introduction

The microscopic study of cells obtained from organs, in the form of serous effusions from cavities or brushings, began in the middle of the 19th century (KOSS, 1972; ACTA, 1998).

George Papanicolaou contributed greatly to the concept of exfoliative cytology using vaginal secretion smears and this concept has been transformed by the use of other techniques to collect cytological samples (EXFOLIATIVE, 1961; MARCONDES, 1975; WIED et al., 1983; OBA, 1988; CORDEIRO et al., 1989; BIBBO, 1991; CARVALHO, 1993; McKEE, 1997).

Cytological examination is a method of diagnostic investigation based on cell morphology acquired through different collection techniques. Any organ can be examined without risk of trauma and with minimal discomfort for the patient (AZÙA, 1976; CORDEIRO et al., 1989; DONAT et al., 1989; DUCATMAN et al., 1989; FRABLE, 1989; GROSS et al., 1992; BRIDGE & ORNDAL, 1999; CURTIS, 2001).

The advantages of cytological examination are well known, as it is a low-cost, simple, outpatient procedure that does not require hospitalization or tranquilizers. It also reduces the need for surgical procedures, whether for unresectable masses or even when surgical treatment is not the first choice (SANDERSON et al, 1980; ROGERS et al, 1996; THOMPSON et al, 1997; MAZETO, 2000; ROCHA et al, 2001a; ROCHA et al, 2001b; SAXE et al, 2001).

Morphological findings can be used to predict the biological behavior of diseases, in an attempt to assess the patient's prognosis (ZACH, 1972; YOUNG, 1994; ZUCCARI, 1999; WHITE, 2000).

The cytopathology test is recognized as being excellent for identifying diseases in humans and animals. However, it is underused when compared to its applicability to humans, as can be seen in scientific articles specializing in the subject (COWELL & TYLER, 1989; COWELL et al., 1999).

Veterinary medical professionals should invest in cytological examination, mainly because it speeds up diagnosis at a low cost. These characteristics benefit the professional's conduct, since certain compulsory diseases can be identified quickly (DOMINGUES et al., 1999; RIBEIRO et al., 2002).

The relevance of the evaluation lies in the speed with which the diagnosis is obtained, unlike the histological technique which requires a few days to properly prepare the material (ZACH,

1972; BAKER & LUMSDEN, 2000; COWELL & TYLER, 2002).

Based on the above considerations, the main objective of this work was to standardize inflammatory and non-inflammatory lesions by cytological examination, in order to add information that can be used to help diagnose animal diseases in the routine of the UNESP Botucatu Veterinary Hospital.

2. Literature

2.1 Laboratory Operating Rules for Cytological Tests

In Brazil, in 1985, the Pan American Health Organization, the World Health Organization and the Ministry of Health carried out a diagnosis of the situation of cytopathology and histopathology laboratories that support the basic health network. The resulting document identified and presented difficulties ranging from the availability of physical, material, human and financial resources to the training and qualification of staff by professional level. This led to the need to draw up a manual to help standardize and unify diagnoses, as well as guiding the installation of laboratories for cytological and histological diagnosis (CUNHA, 1987).

The cytology laboratory complies with state and federal regulations, which require the laboratory to carry out at least 50,000 cytological examinations of the female genital system, cervix and breast, and other systems each year; an annual report on the activities carried out; continuous retraining of the professional staff and periodic evaluations aimed at guaranteeing the quality of the examinations carried out (CUNHA, 1987; KEEBLER & SOMRAK, 1993).

Reports issued by cytopathology laboratories should indicate diagnostic and prognostic parameters that provide sufficient support for the best patient care (DeMAY, 1995; BOLETIM, 2002).

The National Institute of Metrology, Standardization and Industrial Quality, IMETRO, a Federal Autarchy, the executive body of the National System of Metrology, Standardization and Industrial Quality - SINMETRO, has developed a quality certification model for laboratories, in accordance with resolution no.[2] 9 of 24.08.92 (JORNAL, 1997).

GLP (Good Laboratory Practice) are standards that concern the organization and conditions under which studies are planned, carried out, monitored, recorded and reported. In determining their scope, it is clear that they are intended to regulate laboratories related to human, animal and plant health and the environment (EXFOLIATIVE, 1961; CUNHA, 1987).

On the other hand, the International Academy of Cytology considers an experienced professional to be one who has carried out at least 200 tests in a few months and continues to carry out one to two tests a day (EXFOLIATIVE, 1961; CUNHA, 1987).

2.2 Cytological examination

Cytological examination, an important and fundamental tool for identifying normal and diseased cells, first appeared with Papanicolaou (EXFOLIATIVE, 1961).

Despite criticisms and limitations, as an laboratory method, at first exclusively for humans and later used for other animals, it helps to track various forms of lesoes, identifying potentially fatal cases and reducing the impact of those that could cause irreversible diseases (EXFOLIATIVE, 1961; MARCONDES, 1975; JORNAL, 1997; BOLETIM, 2002).

In countries where uterine cancer prevention programs, based on Pap smears, have been carried out in a continuous and disciplined manner, the prevalence rates of the disease have decreased dramatically (CUNHA, 1987, KEEBLER & SOMRAK, 1993).

When cytological samples are collected and fixed properly, even in offices and/or outpatient clinics, they provide material for cytomorphological, immunocytochemical and nucleic acid research using molecular biology methods such as hybrid capture, among others (KOSS, 1972; KEEBLER & SOMRAK, 1993; MAMPRIM, 1999; ZUCCARI, 1999).

Mills, in 1984, considered cytological examination to be a procedure with low operating costs, minimal injection, no need for anesthesia and fast and reliable results in most cases, allowing the clinician to confirm or exclude his suspicion at the time of consultation (DOMINGUES, 1999; DOMINGUES et al.,1999; RIBEIRO et al., 2002).

According to MEYER (1996), the success of cytology depends on the various phases of the technique, from obtaining the sample, preparing the slide to reading it. Difficulties in one or more steps of the technique can affect the results obtained. Even if they don't conclude the diagnosis, cytological examinations can demonstrate their value, describing, for example, the lesion in sufficient detail for immediate surgery, in the case of the presence of malignant tumor characteristics (EMMEL et al., 1964; KOSS, 1972; KOSS et al., 1984; CARVALHO; 1993).

Some studies have shown that, although cytological examination as a diagnostic resource in veterinary practice began in the 1930s, the only factor that discourages the use of this procedure is the small number of professionals qualified in collecting, preparing and interpreting the results (ROSZEL, 1975 apud OBA, 1988).

2.3 The Cell

With regard to the requirements for cytomorphological interpretation, a brief review of the nucleus and cytoplasm of eukaryotic cells, exclusively somatic cells, will be presented.

Living cells today are classified as either prokaryotic or eukaryotic. Despite having a relatively simple structure, prokaryotes are biochemically versatile and diverse: for example, all the main metabolic pathways are found in bacteria, including the three processes for obtaining energy: glycolysis, respiration and photosynthesis (KOSS, 1972; MACLEOD, 1981; BIBBO, 1991; KEEBLER & SOMRAK, 1993; ALBERTS et al., 1997; FARAH, 1997).

Eukaryotic cells, on the other hand, are larger and more complex than prokaryotic cells and contain a larger amount of DNA, along with components that allow the DNA to be processed in a very elaborate way. The DNA of the eukaryotic cell is contained in a membranous nuclear structure, while the cytoplasm contains a variety of organelles also contained in membranes, including mitochondria, which are responsible for the oxidation of molecules derived from food, and, in plants, chloroplasts are directly responsible for photosynthesis (KOSS, 1972; MACLEOD, 1981; BIBBO, 1991; KEEBLER & SOMRAK, 1993; ALBERTS et al, 1997; FARAH, 1997; ZAKHOUR & WELLS, 1999).

Mitochondria and chloroplasts are almost certainly direct descendants of prokaryotic cells that established themselves as internal symbionts in a primordial anaerobic cell (KOSS, 1972; MACLEOD, 1981; BIBBO, 1991; KEEBLER & SOMRAK, 1993; ALBERTS et al., 1997).

Eukaryotic cells are also unique in structures such as the cytoskeleton of filamentous proteins, which, as well as helping to organize the cytoplasm, is responsible for cell movement (KOSS, 1972; MACLEOD, 1981; BIBBO, 1991; KEEBLER & SOMRAK, 1993; ALBERTS et al., 1997; FARAH, 1997).

Of unknown function, the fibrous lamina contributes to the prominence of the nuclear envelope seen in light microscopy, especially in neoplastic cells (MACLEOD, 1981; KEEBLER & SOMRAK, 1993).

The space between the two nuclear membranes - the perinuclear cisterna - is variable and can increase considerably after various injuries, including radiation and inflammation. They are detected in the form of isolated or continuous vacuoles adjacent to the nucleus. The latter is called a perinuclear halo (ZACH, 1972; KEEBLER & SOMRAK, 1993; McKEE, 1997).

Among the nuclear components, chromatin represents the largest percentage, taking up between 25% and 28% of the nuclear volume. Chromatin is made up of 14% to 17% DNA, and the other components are proteins and RNA. Regardless of the variation that occurs during the cell cycle, there is a considerable tendency for chromatin to change its state of distribution in the nuclear compartment, in terms of expansion and contraction. Expansion, the normal form of chromatin presentation in the contracting nucleus, is the altered state. The imbalance in the concentration of calcium and magnesium ions found in the vast majority of diseases, including neoplastic ones, plays a fundamental role in this context (MACLEOD, 1981; KEEBLER & SOMRAK, 1993; FARAH, 1997).

DNA is the carrier of genetic information and is therefore responsible for the cell's properties and abilities. Gene activation and repression are often determined by proteins that also act to maintain DNA integrity. Certain proteins can repair DNA alterations, while others can remove them, preserving genetic integrity. The two main categories of nuclear proteins are histones and non-histones. In cancer cells, there is an enrichment of non-histone acidic proteins, which represent a major factor in nuclear hyperchromasia (MACLEOD, 1981; KEEBLER & SOMRAK, 1993; FARAH, 1997).

The nucleus of a normal egg cell contains the chromosomes from the fusion of the sperm and egg, and is therefore diploid. Alterations in the number of chromosomes and the amount of DNA are called aneuploidies or heteroploidies. Senile cells are more likely to delay mitotic cycles, which can result in an increase in the amount of DNA and consequently in the creation of multiple diploid cells (MACLEOD, 1981; KEEBLER & SOMRAK, 1993; ALBERTS et al., 1997; FARAH, 1997).

The normal cell seen by the exfoliative technique has a round to ovoid nucleus. On the other hand, when errors occur in the genetic material, the nucleus of this cell is phenotypically altered (KOSS, 1972; WIED et al., 1983; KEEBLER & SOMRAK, 1993; McKEE, 1997).

2.4 Spontaneous and Induced Exfoliative Cytology

The tissues lining cavity walls generally consist of four cell layers: basal, parabasal, intermediate and superficial. The latter is made up of older cells which flake off naturally or by means of techniques and can be stained and examined under the microscope (MARCONDES, 1975; KURMAN & SOLOMON, 1994).

The microscopic study of cells obtained from various organs in the form of serous effusions from cavities, sputum and tissue scrapings began in the middle of the 19th century. Although the idea of diagnosing diseases by cytological preparation had already been broached by Europeans, it was George Papanicolaou who brought it into routine use on a large scale (CUNHA, 1987; CARVALHO, 1993; ALVES, 2001).

Cytological samples obtained by printing have proved to be an important screening method, capable of helping in the differential diagnosis of infectious and neoplastic diseases

(LAVACH et al., 1977; PARIDAENS et al., 1992; NOLAN et al., 1994; BAKER & LUMSDEN, 2000; FARIAS, 2000; WHITE, 2000; ROCHA et al., 2001a; SCOTT et al., 2001).

The use of exfoliative cytology as a diagnostic method in veterinary practice has progressed and its systematic use for different diseases affecting animals is a current trend (OBA, 1988; COWELL et al., 1999; WHITE, 2000; COWELL & TYLER, 2002).

Exfoliative cytology as a diagnostic method provides good results, particularly for lesions of the uterine cervix, bronchial mucosa and bladder. In view of this, clinicians can safely institute therapy for the respective lesions (DeMAY et al., 1995; MORRISON, 1998; ALVES, 2001).

The cells obtained by scraping and printing can also be used to assess diseases of the cornea and ocular conjunctiva. Cytological examination to evaluate mare endometritis has achieved excellent applicability as it is a quick, non-invasive and accurate method (TSENG, 1985; PARIDAENS et al., 1992; WHITE, 2000; ROCHA et al., 2001a; COWELL & TYLER, 2002).

Naturally or artificially released breast cells are valuable in the diagnosis of certain diseases, especially cystic ones. To obtain them by ambulatory maneuver, slight pressure on the base of the breast towards the nipple gives good results, when used correctly (AZÙA, 1976; DeMAY, 1995; McKEE, 1997).

2.5 Cytology With and Without Aspiration

Cytological examination with and without aspiration was developed with the aim of treating sites inaccessible to exfoliation (KOSS et al., 1984; MAIR et al., 1989; ACTA, 1998; SUEN, 1990 apud TOSTES,1998).

Aspiration puncture has therefore become an important method for diagnosing diseases in different organs. Initially performed with a high-caliber needle, over the years it has come to be performed with a fine needle, known as fine needle aspiration. This is defined as a diagnostic method which aims to obtain material from a lesion using a needle with an external diameter of 0.6 to 0.9 mm and a length of 1.0 to 20.0 cm (KOSS et al., 1984; MEYER, 1996). As early as the 10th century, an Arab physician used it for diagnostic purposes to distinguish between different types of goiter (KOSS et al., 1984; SILVERMAN et al., 1989). Later, Kun used the same methodology to diagnose tumors (FRABLE, 1989; MOONEY et al., 1995; STERN et al., 2001).

In Brazil, the first publications on aspiration cytology appeared in 1978. Since then, it has developed greatly, proving to be safe, non-invasive and highly accurate in diagnosis, reducing surgical indications and operative complications. As a result, it has become routine in several medical and veterinary institutions (ROCHA et al., 1998; ROCHA et al., 2001b).

Different studies have proven the method's efficiency in certain diagnostic situations compared to other traditional techniques, such as histopathology (KOSS, 1972; TOSTES, 1998).

Recent research in Brazil has successfully used cytology in the presumptive diagnosis of certain infectious diseases in domestic animals. Alternatively, material from different lesions has made it possible to isolate and characterize algae, fungi and bacteria (GREENE, 1990; DOMINGUES, 1999; DOMINGUES et al., 1999; RIBEIRO et al., 2002).

Kumarasinghe (1997) and other authors have referred to cytology as a standardized diagnostic procedure for various breast diseases, including granulomatous mastitis specific to tuberculosis and mycosis (AZÙA, 1976; McKEE, 1997; DOMINGUES, 1999; DOMINGUES et al., 1999).

Since 1981, French authors have modified the aspiration puncture technique to the non-aspiration technique. This method is based on the physical principle that fluid will rise spontaneously in a narrow tube in inverse proportion to its diameter. Thus, the technique is based on inserting the needle into the lesion without connecting it to the syringe and, consequently, without the negative pressure to aspirate the material (LIMA et al., 1988; MAIR et al., 1989; KATE et al., 1998).

Both the puncture with aspiration and the one without are capable of tracing the lesion in an expansion of ten planes or more in relation to the biopsy (DeMAY, 1995; ROCHA, 1998), as well as minimizing the risk of tumor spread (ZAJDELA et al., 1987; KABUKÇUOGLU et al., 1998; ROCHA et al., 2000; ROCHA et al., 2001a).

2.6 Cytology Sample Preparation

The cytological samples are spread out on histological slides, fixed immediately with 95% ethanol or spray fixatives, every time they are to be subjected to Pap, Shorr or hematoxylin and eosin staining. To make better use of the sample, the bevel of the needle can be washed with 50% ethanol. When Romanovisk stains are used, the sample should be dried at room temperature and then fixed with 100% methanol. The choice of cytological sample preparation is determined by the initial clinical inquiry (KOSS et al., 1984; HAJDU, 1989; COWELL & TYLER, 1989).

The number of slides per patient depends on the type and characteristics of the lesion. For breast samples, for example, a minimum of three slides should be processed. For the liver, on the other hand, 10 to 12 slides should be processed when possible; for cystic lesions, the material should be cytocentrifuged for subsequent slide preparation. Cytological samples can be sent for processing to a distant laboratory, as long as the sample is properly fixed (KOSS et al., 1984; HAJDU, 1989).

In the case of cytological diagnosis of neoplasms, although relatively simple, their classification can be difficult. Electron microscopy, immunocytochemistry, among other methodologies, can greatly help the accuracy of diagnosis and add new horizons to cytological practice (HAJDU, 1989; KEEBLER & SOMRAK, 1993).

2.7 Nomenclature for Cytopathological Examination Reports

After Papanicolaou introduced the basics of diagnosing malignancy using exfoliative cytology, progress in the fight against cancer evolved worldwide. Although the idea of diagnosing neoplasms through the use of cytological preparations had already been addressed by some European researchers, it was Papanicolaou who put it into practice, with routine use on a large scale (MARCONDES, 1975; CARVALHO, 1993).

Initially almost restricted to the diagnosis of cervical cancer, cytology today extends to all areas of human and animal anatomy, with such firmness and precision that to many it may seem an exaggeration to speak of precancerous lesions or invasive tumors (MARCONDES, 1975; CARVALHO, 1993; KURMAN & SOLOMON, 1994).

In 1993, the Brazilian Society of Cytopathology, with the support of the Ministry of Health, through the National Cancer Institute, drew up and later made official the first Brazilian nomenclature for uterine cervical cytopathology reports. This standardization applied in Brazil was enshrined in the "Viva Mulher Program" from 1995 onwards (CUNHA, 1987; BOLETIM, 2002).

In 2001, eight years had passed during which new technologies and new morphological and molecular knowledge had emerged, including the revision of the Bethesda System. The Brazilian Society of Pathology and the Ministry of Health were actively involved (CUNHA, 1987; KURMAN & SOLOMON, 1994; BOLETIM, 2002).

The National Cancer Institute, the Ministry of Health and the Brazilian Society of Cytopathology brought together their professionals and revised the nomenclature, with the contribution and participation of pathologists, cytologists and the Brazilian Society of Pathology. After extensive discussion, the following structure was defined: a) type of sample - conventional cytology and liquid cytology; b) pre-analytical assessment - rejected material; c) adequacy of the sample - satisfactory and unsatisfactory; d) descriptive diagnosis

(CUNHA, 1987; BOLETIM, 2002).

The interpretation of cytological samples obtained by puncture, lavage, expression, among others, aims to define neoplastic, degenerative or inflammatory processes. As cytological samples contain cells that are separated from their structural organization, the problem is reduced to the possible existence of morphological alterations that are specific or unspecific to the cell. Therefore, in cytology this search is not based on a single alteration, but on a sum of data (ZACH, 1972; MARCONDES, 1975; CARVALHO, 1993; McKEE, 1997; KOJIMA et al., 1998; ALVES, 2001).

Degenerative changes are common and should be recognized as such. They are observed in the vast majority of neoplastic cells derived from parabasal and sidewalk cells. These changes include an increase in cell volume; with a change in the staining pattern and a loss of sharpness of the nuclear boundaries (EXFOLIATIVE, 1961; KOSS, 1972; ZACH, 1972; McKEE, 1997).

Inflammation is the form of tissue reaction to an injury. There are four main types of inflammation: acute, subacute, chronic and granulomatous. These processes are easily recognized in the cytological sample. Acute inflammation is characterized by necrosis and tissue exhaustion. The predominant inflammatory cell is the neutrophil. On the other hand, in subacute inflammation, tissue damage is less severe, but the duration is much longer than in acute inflammation and eosinophils and lymphocytes are the predominant cells (EXFOLIATIVE, 1961; KOSS, 1972; ZACH, 1972; MARCONDES, 1975; McKEE, 1997).

Chronic inflammation results in mild tissue aggression, offset by repair. The lymphocyte is the most prominent cell, with the occasional plasma cell, histiocyte and/or macrophage. Granulomatous inflammation is a variant of chronic inflammation, characterized by a cluster of histiocytic cells reminiscent of epithelial cells, multinucleated giant cells and lymphocytes (KOSS, 1972; ZACH, 1972; MARCONDES, 1975; McKEE, 1997; BAKER & LUMSDEN, 2000; COWELL & TYLER, 2002).

None of the cellular alterations alone constitute an absolutely reliable criterion for diagnosing lesions. However, proof of several criteria and the frequency with which they manifest themselves are convincing and reliable arguments in the cytological observation of the examined material (KOSS, 1972; ZACH, 1972; MARCONDES, 1975; CARVALHO, 1993; McKEE, 1997; ROCHA et al., 2001b).

3. Objective

To date, there has been no similar study in national veterinary medicine.

In view of the need to acquire extensive knowledge about the use of cytological examination in veterinary practice, this study was developed with the aim of recording inflammatory and non-inflammatory lesions in animals and including cytopathology in the list of auxiliary techniques used in the Veterinary Pathology Service at the UNESP Veterinary Hospital in Botucatu.

4. Material and Methods

4.1 Cytopathology at UNESP Botucatu Veterinary Hospital

The standardization of the cytological examination technique followed the norms established for Cytopathology Laboratories by the Pan American Health Organization, the World Health Organization, the Ministry of Health and adaptations made by the Veterinary Pathology Service - UNESP Botucatu. From that moment on, the Department of Veterinary Clinics and later other Departments of FMVZ - UNESP and the Hospital's supervision became aware of it and, in March 1994, approved its use in the routine care of the Surgery, Dermatology, Reproduction, Infectious Diseases and Large and Small Animal Surgery and Reproduction Centers of the Veterinary Hospital of the Faculty of Veterinary Medicine and Zootechnics of UNESP, Botucatu Campus.

4.1.1 Patient Inclusion Criteria

From March 1994 to June 2002, we included animals of different species, breeds, sexes and ages seen at the various facilities of the Veterinary Hospital of the Faculty of Veterinary Medicine and Zootechny - UNESP, for medical treatment. The animals which, after physical assessment, showed lesions on the skin, subcutaneous tissue, apparent mucous membranes and closed cavities, and bones were submitted to cytological examination (Figure 5).

Four groups were formed according to species, sex, age group (0-5; 6-10; 11-15 and 16-20 years) and lesion topography (superficial and deep): Group 1, animals with lesions in the skin and subcutaneous region (Figure 5c); Group 2, animals with lesions in the external mucosa (Figures 5a and b); Group 3, animals with lesions in the bone and closed cavity (Figures 5d and e); Group 4, animals with cavity fluid (Figure 5f). In the latter, the material was collected in the clinic.

For groups 1 and 2, when it wasn't possible to pinpoint the exact extent of the lesion by palpation, imaging (radiography and ultrasound) was used; for group 3, the use of imaging became mandatory.

4.1.2 Collection Technique for Cytological Examination in the Outpatient Clinic and Surgical Center

Before collecting the cytological sample from the animals in each group, they were individually identified on a standardized request form from the Pathology department, which contained all the information needed for the cytological examination. In addition, the person responsible for the patient signed an Informed Consent form, stating that they were aware of the possible risks of the examination for the animal. This was optional for Groups 1 and 2 and mandatory for Group 3 (Figures 1 and 2).

Figura 1 -Requisition **sheet** for identification, collection and diagnosis of cytological examination. **Rocha, 1994**. Adaptation

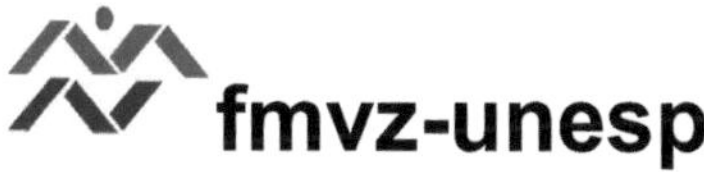

FACULTY OF VETERINARY MEDICINE AND ZOOTECHNY - BOTUCATU

VETERINARY HOSPITAL - PATHOLOGY SERVIÇO

CITOLOGIA

CEP 18.618-000 - Cx Postal 560 - Botucatu - SP - Rubiao Jr. - PBX (014) 6820-6293 - FAX 6820-6067

Registration № Cytology № Specify:

Owner:

Address:

Species: Breed: Sex: Age: -----------------------------

Requester: --

Signature:

Summary, suspicion, clinic and map of the lesion:

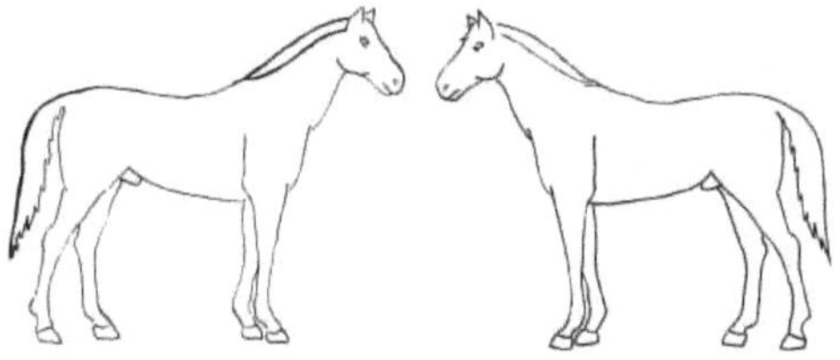

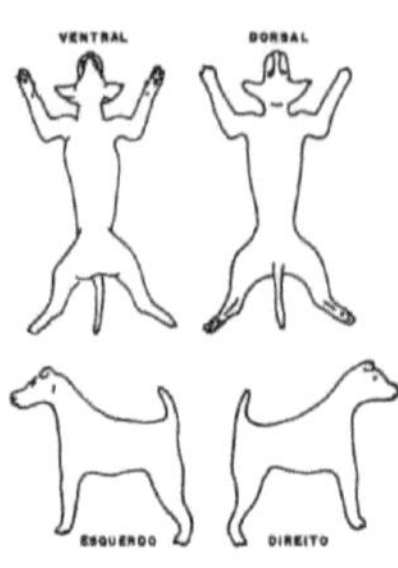

Type of fixation: Coloring:

Adequacy of the sample:

Adequacy of the sample:

Satisfactory Satisfactory but limited Unsatisfactory

Specify:

Diagnosis:infamatio O non-inflammatory O

Specify

Descriptive / Conclusive:

Date: ___ / ___ / ___

Cytologist

Figura 2 - Free and informed consent form. **Rocha, 1994**.

I hereby inform you that I am aware and fully aware that the procedure may pose risks to the animal, whose

responsibility is entirely mine.

Name: RG: --

Signature: Place and date: -------------------

The methods used to collect the cell samples were: cytology with aspiration (CCA), cytology without aspiration (CSA), spontaneous exfoliative cytology (CEE) and induced exfoliative cytology (IEC).

CSA, CCA and CEI were used on the lesions of Group 1 animals. CSA was used for lesions up to 1 cm in diameter. For lesions above this diameter, CCA was used. For breasts with secretion, the CCI was used, by expression.

The material used in the CCA was a 10ml disposable syringe with 26G ½ (13x4.5mm), 22G

(30x7mm) and 25G (90x5mm) disposable needles, the latter exclusively for Group 3, and a Valeri Cytoaspirator (Figures 6c and e).

The CCA was applied as follows: the needle was connected to the syringe which, in turn, was coupled to the cytoaspirator. After local antisepsis, the lesion was punctured and negative pressure was applied, repositioning the needle without it leaving the lesion. The negative pressure was then relaxed and the needle removed from the lesion; the syringe was then uncoupled and a sufficient volume of air was drawn into the syringe to expel the contents of the needle onto a histological slide with a frosted tip. The material was immediately extended in one direction using another histological slide (Figures 7a-i).

For the CSA technique, the lesion was immobilized with one hand, while the needle was introduced into the target with the other hand. The needle was moved in different directions inside the tumor. After removing the needle, it was connected to the air-filled syringe and the material was expelled onto the histological slide (Figures 8a-e).

In the process, one hand was used to massage the affected gland from base to apex, similar to milking (Figure 10c). Sometimes, the excretion product acquired by this maneuver was placed directly on a histological slide or was subjected to the same procedure as for effusion and washing, depending on the consistency and quantity of the sample (Figure 6f).

In Group 2, the CEI technique was used. When the lesion was on the external ocular conjunctiva, the material used was regenerated cellulose membrane and/or filter paper (0E67 - 0.45µmx47mm, Schleicher & Schüll). At the site of the lesion, the paper was pressed for two to three seconds and then the sample obtained was carefully transferred to a histological slide with a frosted edge, so as to preserve the identification of the affected area without causing deformities in the cell (Figures 10a and b).

Also in Group 2, whose lesions were on the mucous membranes of the ear, oral or nasal cavity and external genitalia, the material used was: a flexible rod with a cotton tip (cotton bud - Johnson & Johnson), for puppies and/or miniature animals, moistening the cotton with saline solution to prevent the cells from adhering to the cotton, an Ayra spatula (Carl Parker Associates, New York, USA) and a cervical brush (Kolplast), for the other patients (Figure 6b).

When the flexible rod and/or brush was used at the site of the lesion, it was turned five times in one direction and then the sample was placed on the histological slide with a frosted edge in the same direction (Figures 9a and c).

Ayra's spatula was used to collect material exclusively from the oral cavity and external genitalia of the female. On the surface of the lesion, depending on its consistency, it was exfoliated one or more times in the same direction, with the edge of the spatula moistened in physiological solution. The sample obtained was then placed on the histological slide with a frosted edge (Figures 9a and b).

The collection of material by the Group 4 EEC was at the discretion of the outpatient department. It was therefore up to this sector to receive, process and analyze the samples.

4.1.2 Cytological Examination Organization and Processing

4.1.2.1 Receipt of cytology samples by the laboratory

Samples coming in for analysis were recorded in the Log Book and given the Laboratory's identification. Requests that were filled out inappropriately or samples that were not identified were rejected administratively, preventing them from being registered and reports from being issued.

For liquid material, cytocentrifugation was carried out (Cytocentrifuge Ciclo Cito - REVAN, Brazil), rotating at 1.5 to 2 rpm/6 minutes (Figure 6f).

4.1.2.2 Fixation and staining of the cytological examination

The use of a fixative solution was a prerequisite for all the smears, with wet fixation with 100% methanol and absolute ethanol being the most frequently used. Before fixing the slides with methanol, they were kept at room temperature for 5 minutes. For those fixed with ethanol, the procedure was immediate. Depending on the type of fixation, the samples were subjected to Shorr, Giemsa and Diff-Quik staining (Figures 17 and 18). The latter was only used when the sample was from a high-risk patient (emergency room) or to confirm the presence of satisfactory material for diagnosis. Reserve slides were kept for future specific staining and immunohistochemistry, when there was a need to identify the causative agent of the lesion or the cellular origin.

4.1.2.3 Cytological Examination Reading System

The initial checking of the slides was one of the resident's tasks, while the final diagnosis was the responsibility of the teacher.

Initially, the sample was confirmed with the corresponding requisition and the condition of the material was checked under a light microscope. Reading was first carried out with a lower magnification objective (3.2x/10.06), when quality control was carried out on the sample in terms of quantity, thickness, coloring and distribution. Then, using higher magnification lenses (10x/0.20; 20x/0.40; 40x/0.65 and 100x/1.30), all the fields were read.

When the reading was complete, the diagnosis was issued in the form of a report. In general, the reading of each slide took between 5 and 10 minutes (Figure 3).

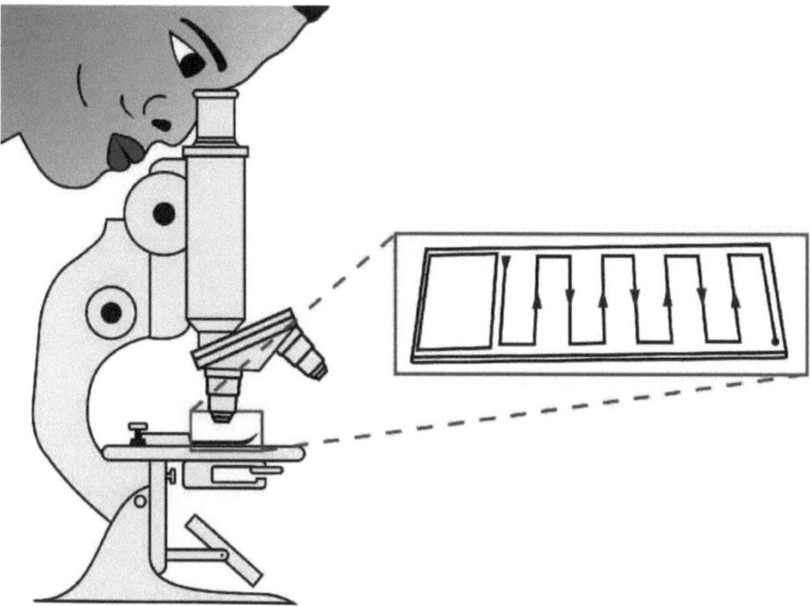

Figure 3 - Technique for reading the cytological sample under the microscope (Carl Zaiss-Jenamed-2 Germany). **Cunha, 1987**.

4.1.2.4 Morphological criteria for diagnosing the cytological examination

The diagnostic criterion used for all groups was based on the predominant cell type, which made it possible to determine whether the process was of an inflammatory or non-inflammatory nature and/or a combination of both. The worldwide agreement to unify the diagnosis with the use of semi-quantitative nomenclature, which was related to histology, prevailed (Figures 4, 11, 12, 13 and 14).

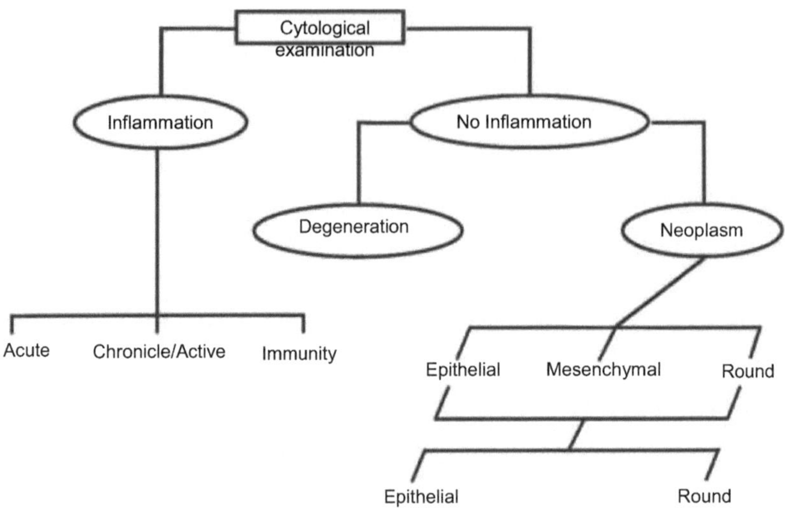

Figure 4 - Nomenclature used in the diagnosis of cytological material. Adapted from: Reppas & Canfield, 1995

4.1.2.5 Inflammatory process - acute, chronic/active, pyogenic - lomatous, granulomatous, immune: specific and non-specific.

The presence of a high number of neutrophils (> 75%) was diagnosed as acute inflammation (Figure 12b). When the proportion of eosinophils was around 10% to 15%, specific diseases such as eosinophilic granuloma complex and mycosis were investigated (Figure 12c). When more than 50% of the cells were macrophages, it was called an inflammatory process of the granulomatous type; however, when there were more than 15% and less than 50% macrophages among a significant population of neutrophils, the process was called pyogranulomatous (Figures 12b and e).

In cases where 15% of macrophages associated with lymphocytes and fibroblasts were detected, the process was identified as chronic/active (Figures 12e 4. Material and Methods and f). The presence of lymphocytes, plasma cells and eosinophils interspersed with 15% macrophages was diagnosed as an immune process (Figures 12f, g, c and e).

Regardless of the type of inflammation, the term specific was added when it was possible to identify the causative agent. Otherwise, unspecific was added (Figures 12a-h).

4.1.2.6 Non-inflammatory process - degenerative, hyperplastic, dysplastic and neoplastic

When the sample contained a large amount of mucoprotein, cholesterol, red blood cells, vacuolization, cell debris, calcium deposition and edema, the process was considered degenerative (hematoma, seroma, hygroma, sialocele, calcinosis and dermoid cyst) (Figures 11c f, 12h and 14a, b, c).

- Hematoma, when the liquid was dark and under the microscope there were activated macrophages, red blood cells and their decomposition products such as hematoidin or hemosiderin crystals and no platelets;

- Seroma and hygroma, when at the time of collection the liquid was transparent and slightly yellowish, with scarce cellularity and composed of macrophage and cyst lining cells;

- Sialocele, when the sample was transparent or reddish viscous and microscopically there was a lake-like secretion and foamy cells (macrophage or degenerated epithelial cell);

- Calcinosis, when the sample was rich in amorphous basophilic material and sometimes showed macrophage, lymphocyte, giant cell and calcium deposition;

- Epidermoid cyst, when the epithelial component of desquamation is extremely cellular and sometimes contains cholesterol.

For the diagnosis of neoplasia, we considered the origin (Figures 11a, b, d and e) and cell morphology (nuclear and cytoplasmic) (Figures 14h-q) and the panoramic arrangement on the slide (cohesive or threshed) (Figures 13a, b and c). With regard to the aggressiveness of benign and malignant tumors, the approach was the predominant cell type with its morphological atypia and arrangement. The sample was considered malignant when, at the end of reading at least three slides, it presented more than three criteria, preferably nuclear. With the exception of breast tumor, when these criteria were interspersed with an inflammatory picture,

The clinician was asked to reduce this process and, after thirty days, the examination was repeated to confirm or exclude the diagnosis of neoplasia.

4.1.2.7 Criteria for Adequate Cytodiagnosis

Three criteria were established for the use of the cytology sample reading in the final diagnostic conclusion: satisfactory for the diagnosis; satisfactory but limited and; unsatisfactory. The sample was considered satisfactory when it met all the requirements of quality control; a satisfactory but limited sample when the requisition (Figure 1) lacked pertinent clinical information or there were no cells and the smear was obscured by 50% to 75% due to drying artifacts, cell overlap, red blood cells; the sample was unsatisfactory when the smear was obscured by more than 75%. For the last two criteria, an explanatory note requested that the test be repeated at a time interval compatible with its purpose.

4.6 Procedure for archiving slides and reports

The file for the slide, request and report followed the World Health Organization standard, which recommends that slides from cytological cases with negative results for neoplasms be filed for two years from the date of collection, and those positive for neoplasms for an indefinite period (Figure 6g). The requests for all the tests with their respective reports should also be filed in the cytopathology laboratory. Consultation of this file for a period of more than 24 hours should only be allowed when requested in writing.

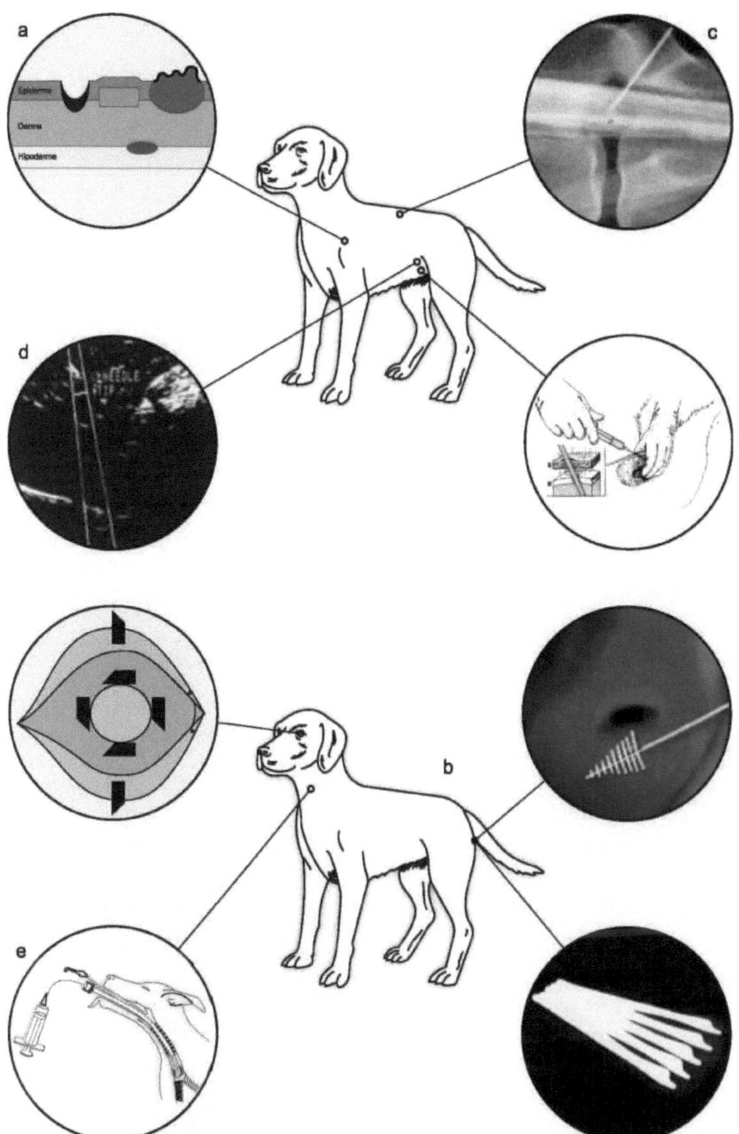

Figure 5 - Group selection.

a - Group 1: cutaneous and subcutaneous lesions; **b** - Group 2: apparent mucous membranes; **c** and **d** - Group 3: closed cavities and bones and **f** - Group 4: serous effusions from closed cavities.

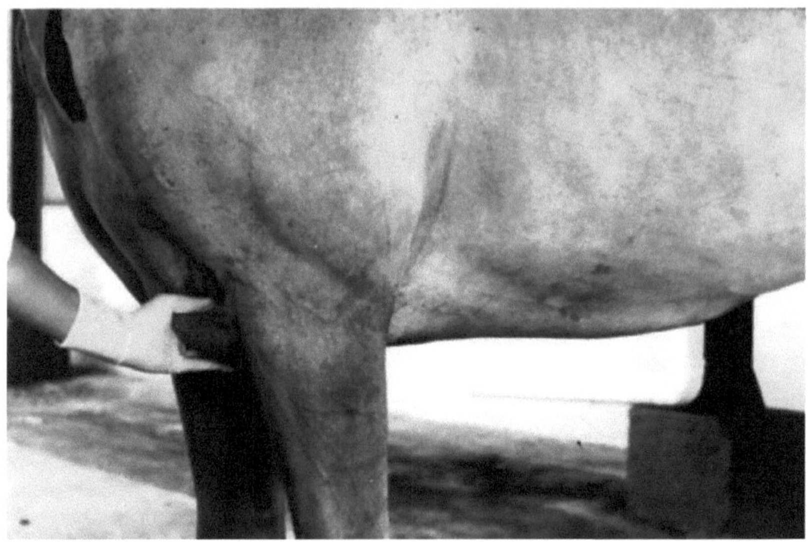

Figure 15 - Equine, physical assessment of the lesion.

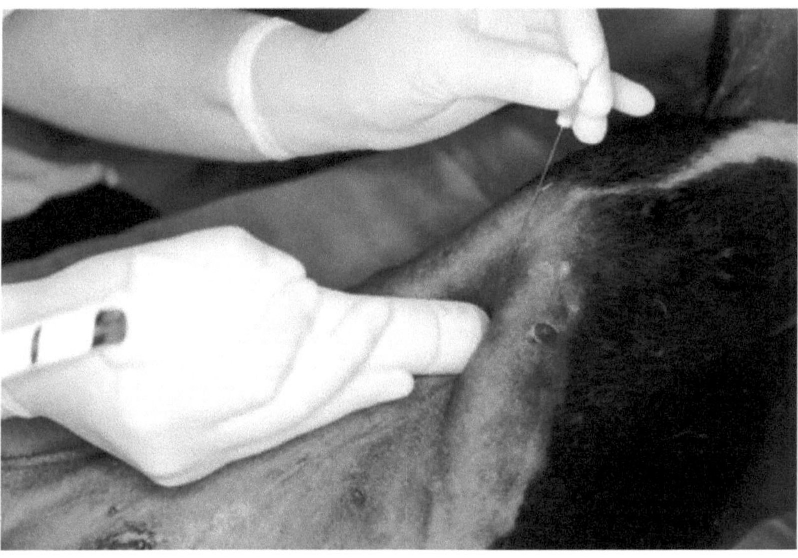

Figure 16 - Ultrasound guiding the collection of cytological samples from the dog's liver.

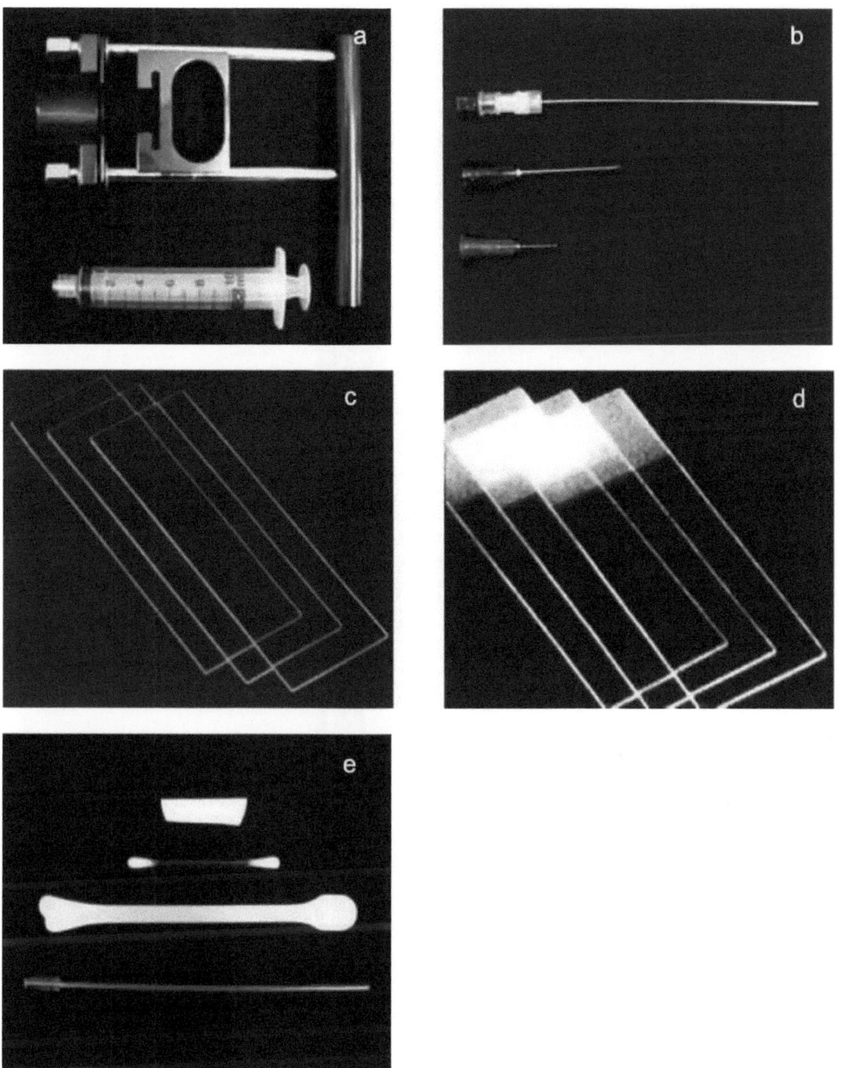

Figure 6 - Material used to collect, process and archive cytological samples **a** - Histological slides with frosted edges; **b** - View from top to bottom: degenerated cellulose membrane, cotton swab, spatula and gynecological brush; **c** - View from top to bottom: Valeri cytoaspirator and 10 ml disposable syringe; **d** - Histological slides without frosted edges; **e** - View from top to bottom: 25G (90x5 mm), 22G (30x7 mm) and 26G ½ (13x4.5 mm) needles; **f** - View from right to left: cytocentrifuge, cytofunnel and filter paper: **g** - slide file.

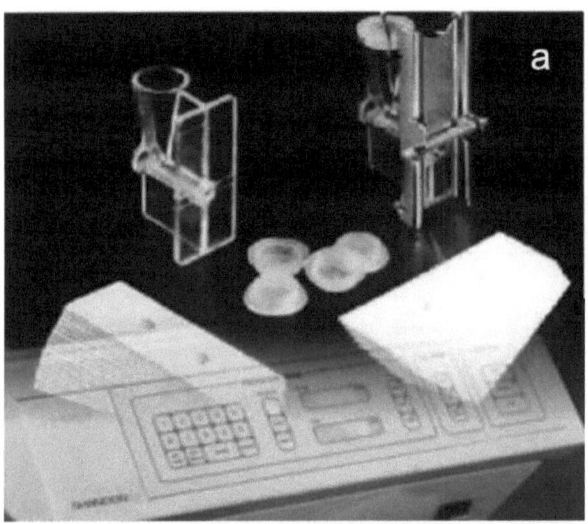

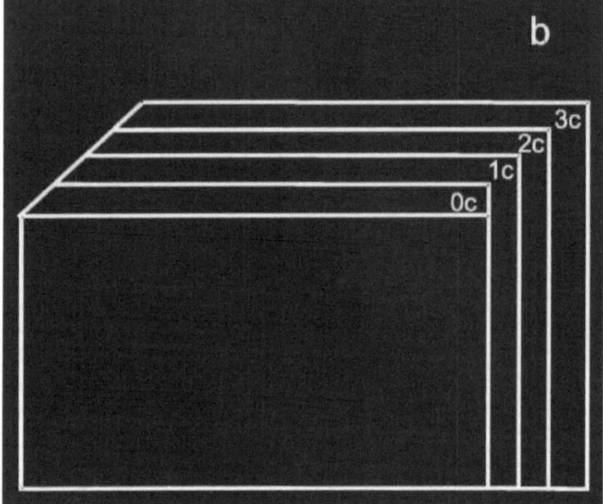

Figure 6 - Material used to collect, process and archive cytological samples **a** - Histological slides with frosted edges; **b** - View from top to bottom: degenerated cellulose membrane, cotton swab, spatula and gynecological brush; **c** - View from top to bottom: Valeri cytoaspirator and 10 ml disposable syringe; **d** - Histological slides without frosted edges; **e** - View from top to bottom: 25G (90x5 mm), 22G (30x7 mm) and 26G ½ (13x4.5 mm) needles; **f** - View from right to left: cytocentrifuge, cytofunnel and filter paper: **g** - slide file.

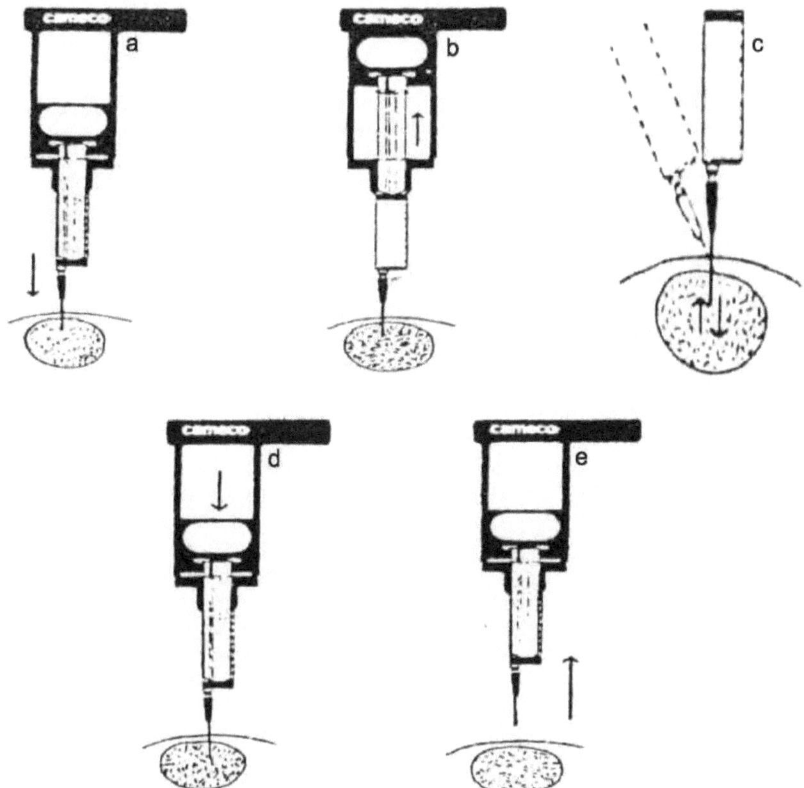

Figure 7 - Collecting the sample from the lesion using the aspiration cytology technique - CCA **a** - Entering the lesion; **b** - Creating negative pressure; **c** - Maintaining negative pressure and directing the needle in a "fan" shape; **d** - Undoing the negative pressure; **e** - Removing the needle from the lesion; **f** - Disconnecting the needle from the syringe; **g** - Aspirating the air into the syringe; **h** - Placing the sample on the histological slide with a frosted edge; **i** - Making the smear.

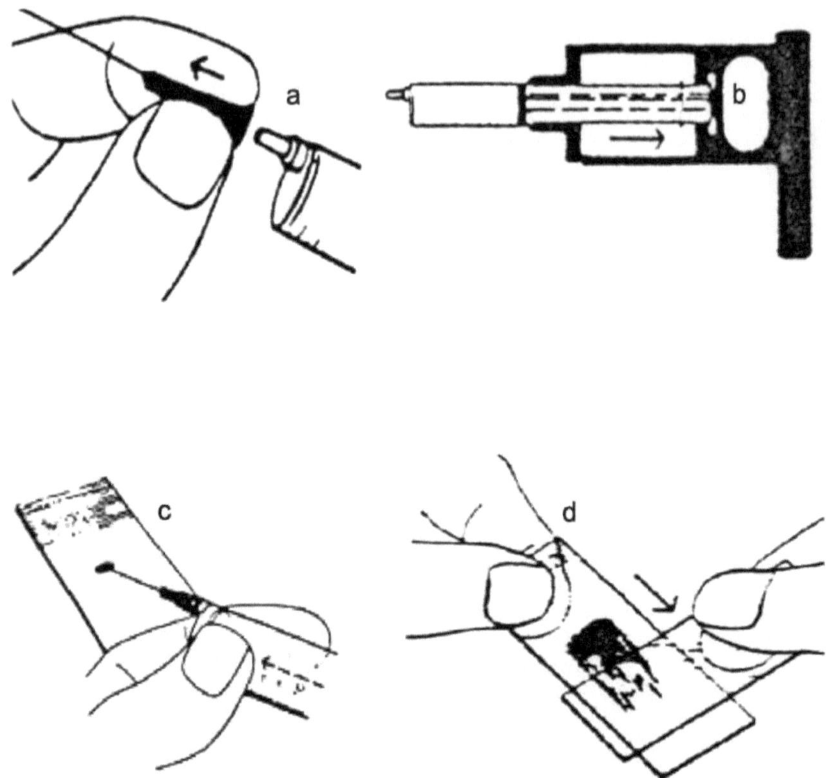

Figure 7 - Collecting the sample from the lesion using the aspiration cytology technique - CCA **a** - Entering the lesion; **b** - Creating negative pressure; **c** - Maintaining negative pressure and directing the needle in a "fan" shape; **d** - Undoing the negative pressure; **e** - Removing the needle from the lesion; **f** - Disconnecting the needle from the syringe; **g** - Aspirating the air into the syringe; **h** - Placing the sample on the histological slide with a frosted edge; **i** - Making the smear.

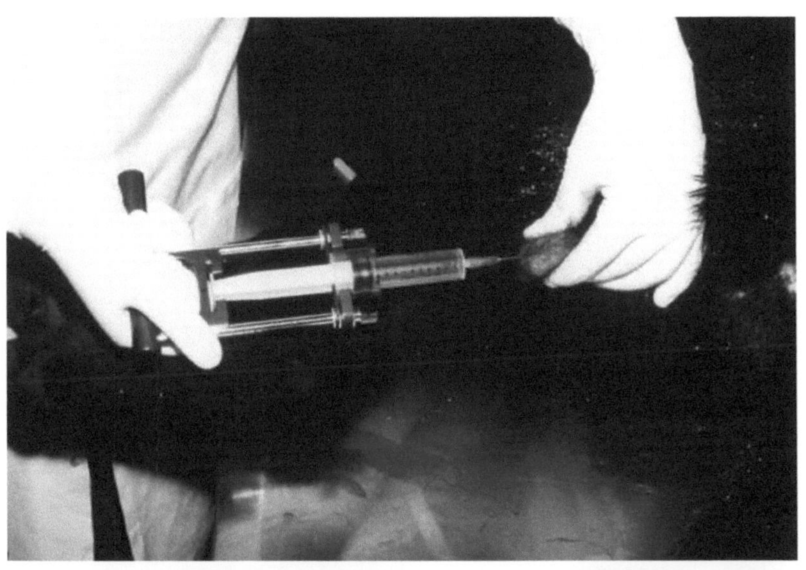

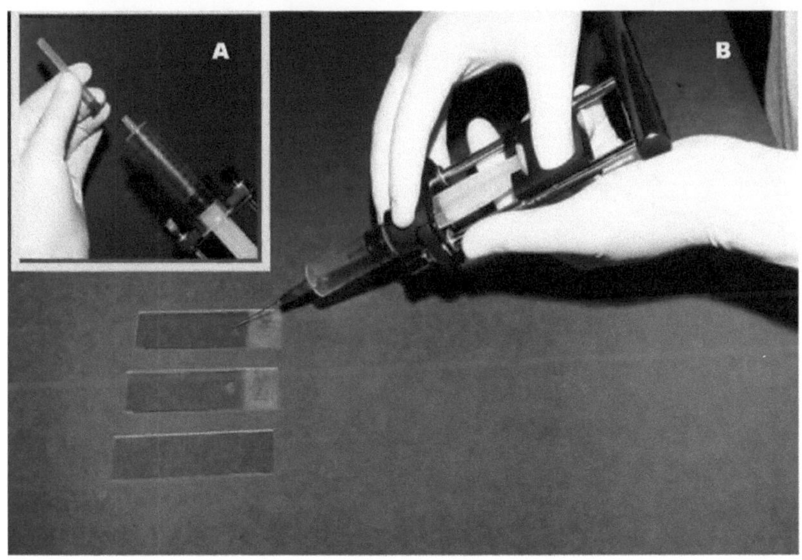
A
B

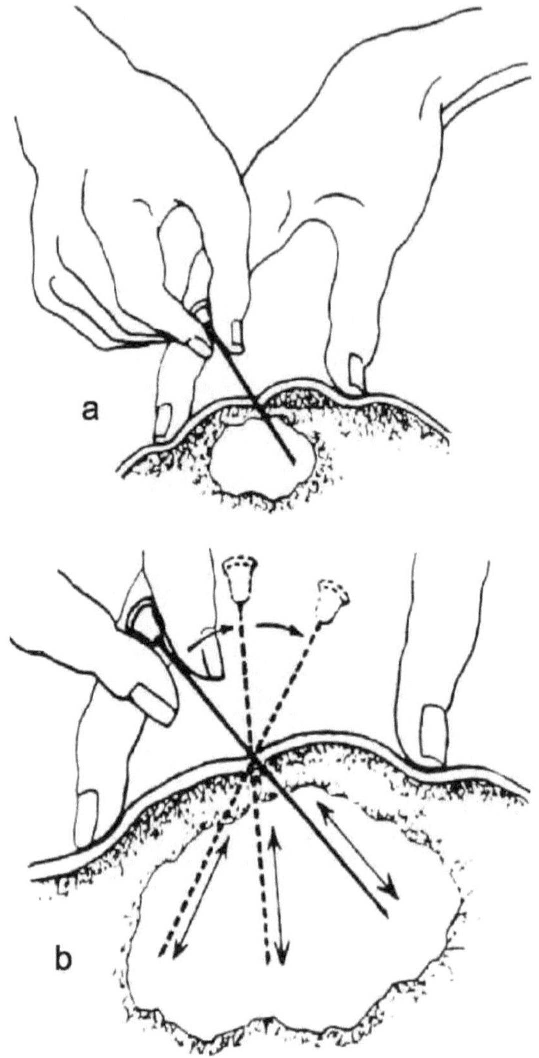

Figure 8 - Collecting a sample from the lesion using the cytology without aspiration technique - CSA

a - Fixing the lesion with one hand and inserting the needle with the other; **b** - Moving the needle inside the mass in various directions; **c** - Connecting the needle to the syringe; **d** - Placing the material on the slide; **e** - Taking the smear.

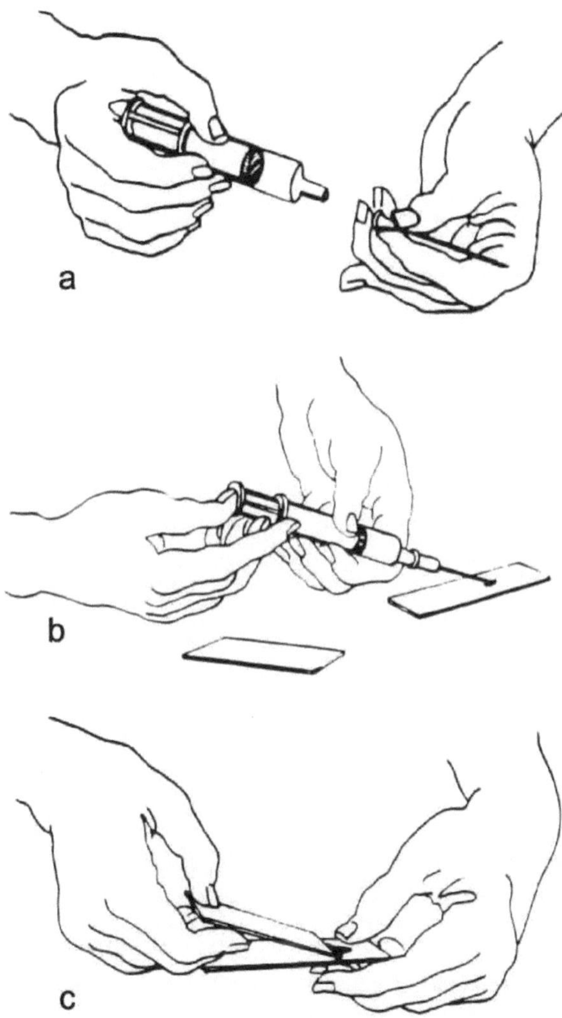

Figura 8 - Collecting a sample from the lesion using the cytology without aspiration technique - CSA

a - Fixing the lesion with one hand and inserting the needle with the other; **b** - Moving the needle inside the mass in various directions; **c** - Connecting the needle to the syringe; **d** - Placing the material on the slide; **e** - Taking the smear.

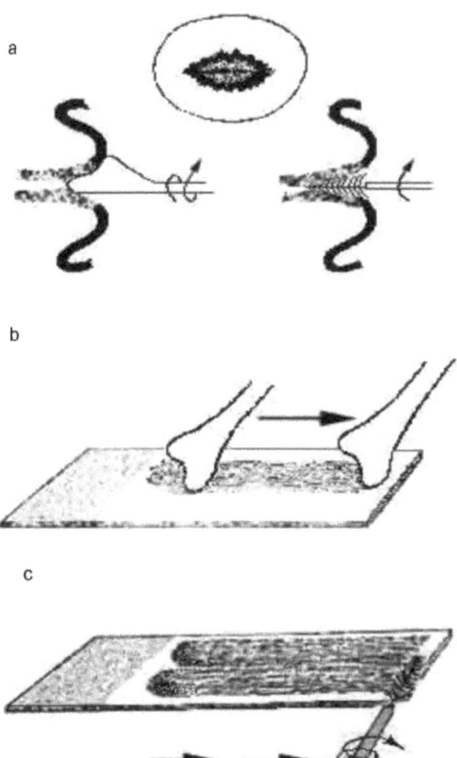

Figura 9 - Collecting a sample of the lesion using the exfoliative cytology technique induced by a spatula or gynecological brush - CEI_1

a - Introducing the spatula or gynecological brush in a single direction into the mucosa; **b and c** - Distending the material in the same direction as the collection on the histological slide with a frosted edge.

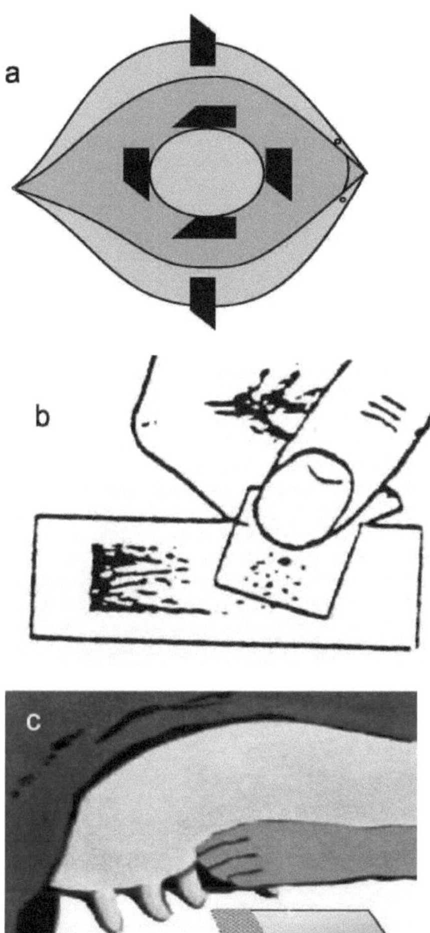

Figura 10 - Sampling of the lesion using the technique of exfoliative cytology induced by imprinting or expression - CEI_2

a - Printing the degenerated cellulose membrane on different areas of the external ocular conjunctiva; **b** - Distending the sample of the lesion on the histological slide with a frosted edge; **c** - Massaging the breast and bringing the histological slide with a frosted edge closer to receive the secretion.

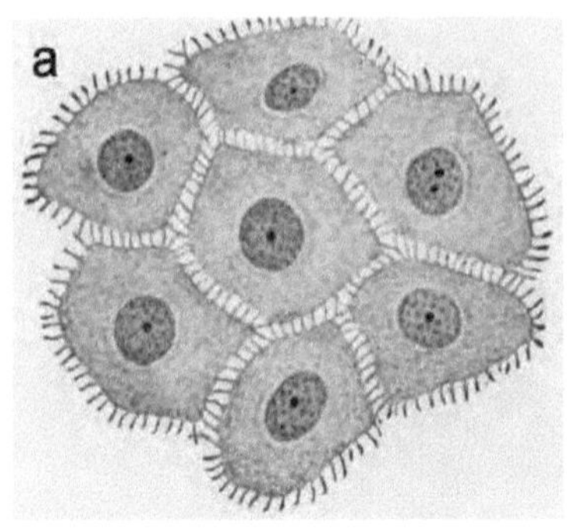

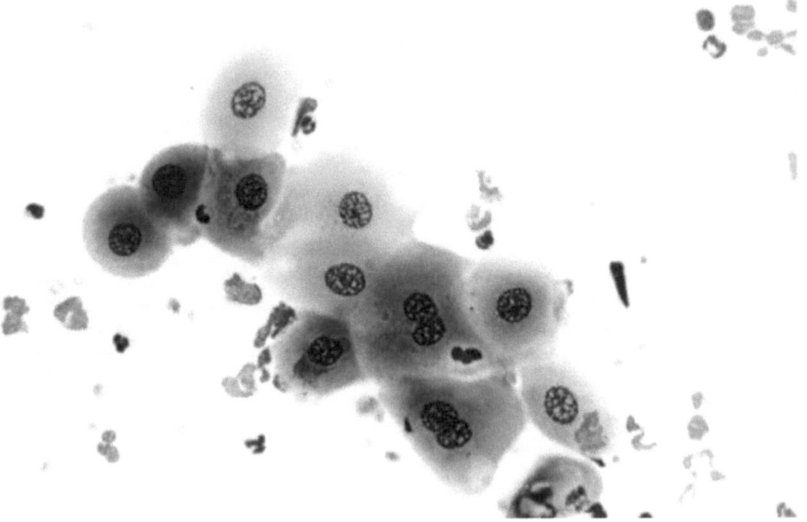

Figura 11 - Criteria used to identify cell origin and secretion products (**Maximow & Bloom, 1942; Esfoliative, 1961; Marcondes, 1975**): - Epithelial cells

Figura 12 - Standardization of the technique and staining of the sample - CEI - regenerated cell membrane. Conjunctiva of the eye. GIEMSA, 40x.

Figura 13

b

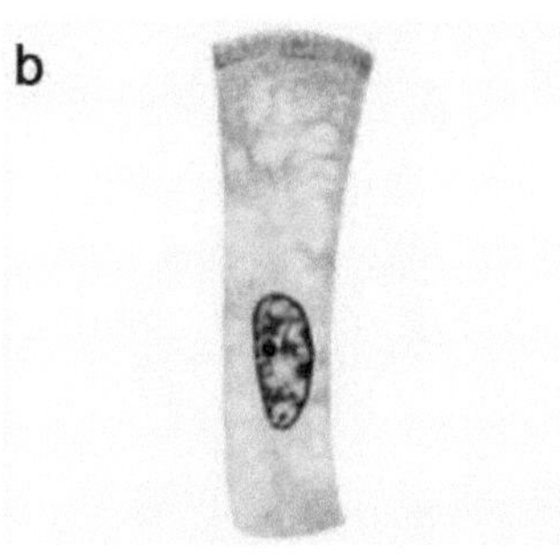

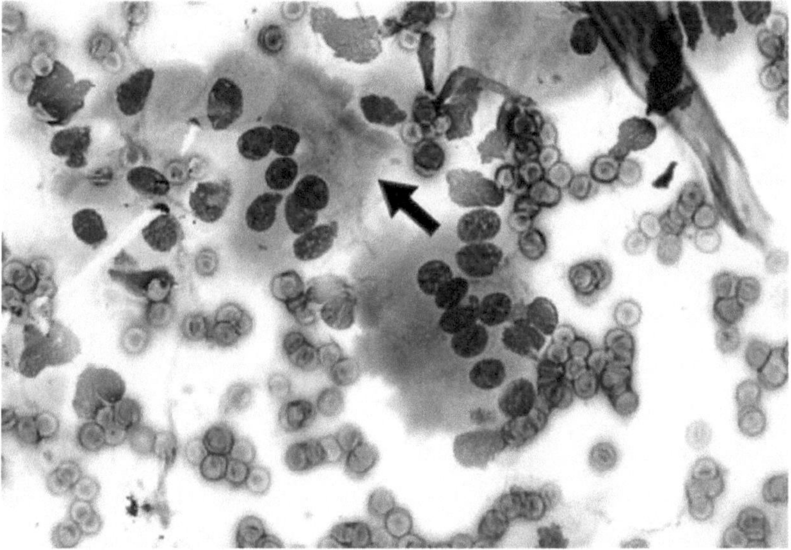

Figure 11 - Criteria used to identify cell origin and secretion products (**Maximow & Bloom, 1942; Esfoliative, 1961; Marcondes, 1975**).

a and b - Epithelial cells; **b and e** - Mesenchymal cells; ; **c** - Mucus; **f** - Cholesterol crystals and **g** - Oxalate crystals.

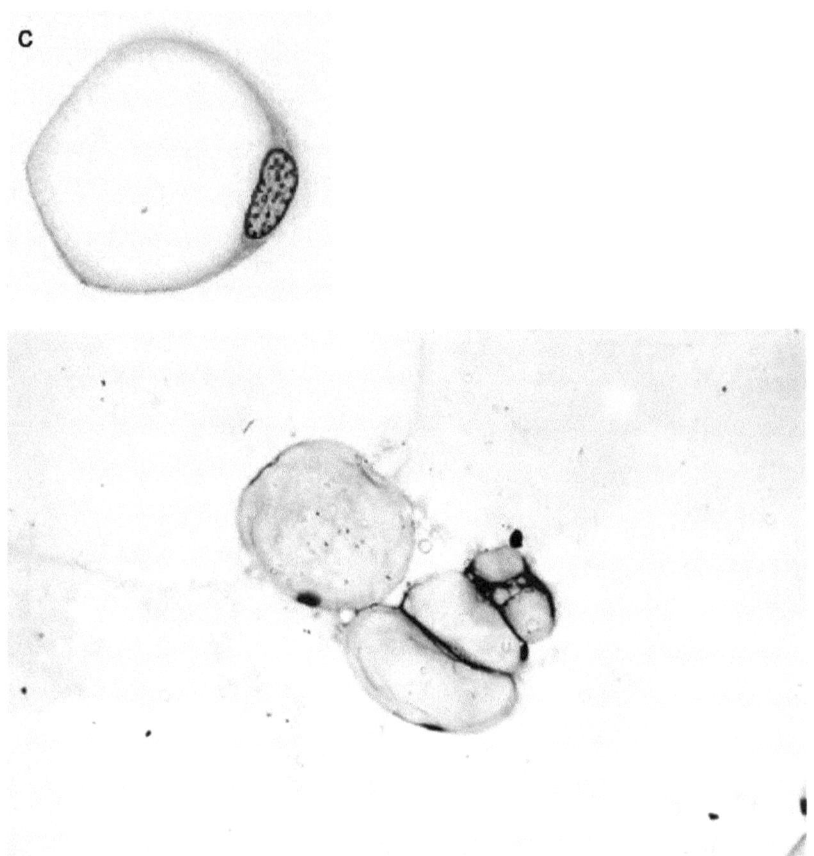

Figure 11 - Criteria used to identify cell origin and secretion products (Maximow **& Bloom, 1942; Esfoliative, 1961; Marcondes, 1975**).

Figure 38 - Feline lipidosis - CCA - fine needle aspiration. Fig. GIEMSA, 40x.

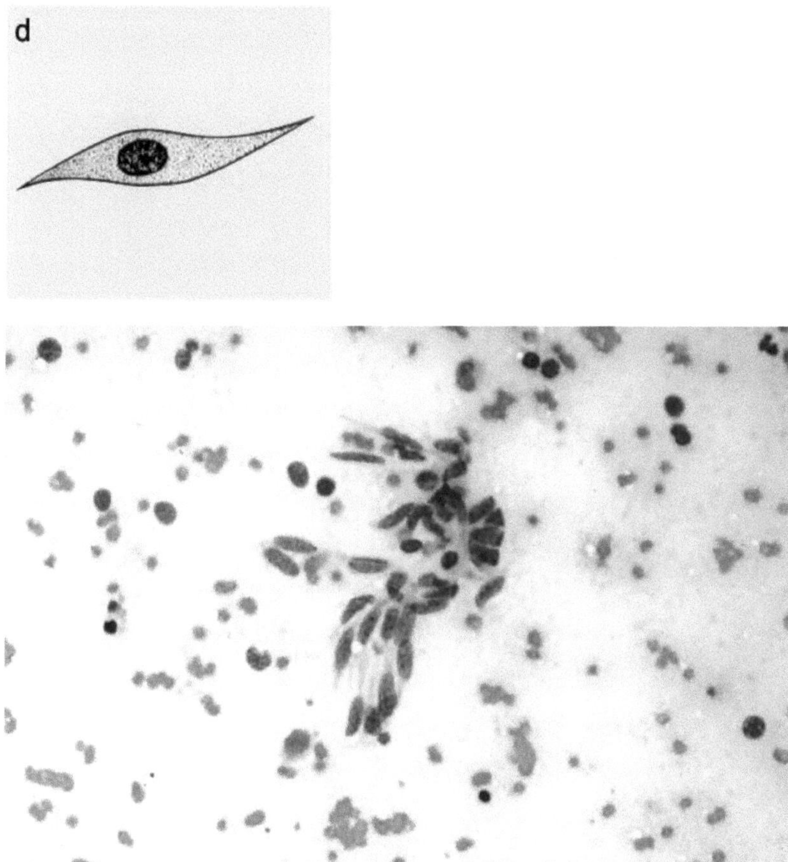

Figure 11 - Criteria used to identify cell origin and secretion products (**Maximow & Bloom, 1942; Esfoliative, 1961; Marcondes, 1975**).

a and b - Epithelial cells; **b and e** - Mesenchymal cells; ; **c** - Mucus; **f** - Cholesterol crystals and **g** - Oxalate crystals.

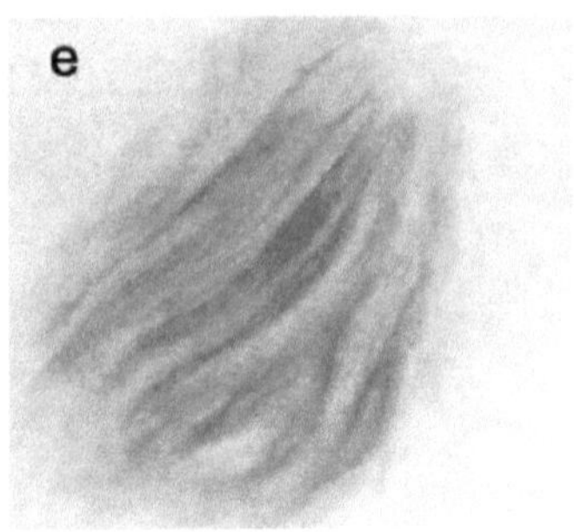

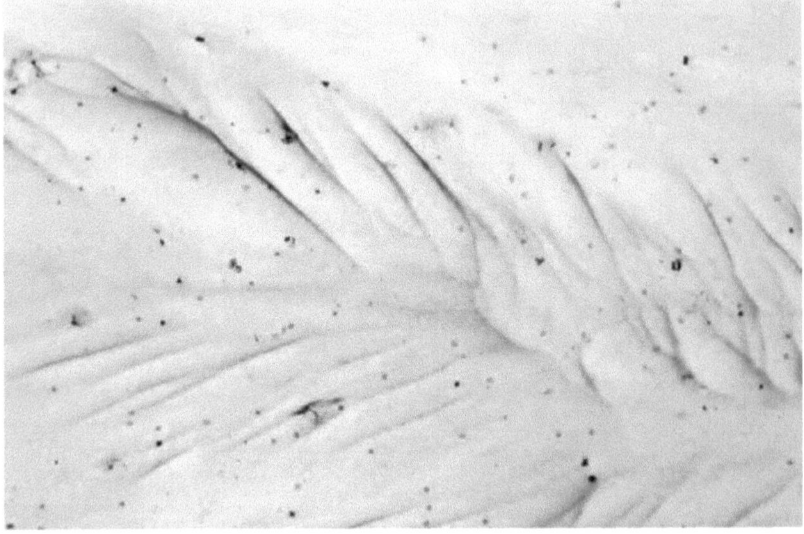

Figure 11 - Criteria used to identify cell origin and secretion products (**Maximow & Bloom, 1942; Esfoliative, 1961; Marcondes, 1975**).

Figure 11 - Hormonal influence of fern-shaped mucin. CEI - gynecological brush. Vagina of a female dog. GIEMSA, 40x.

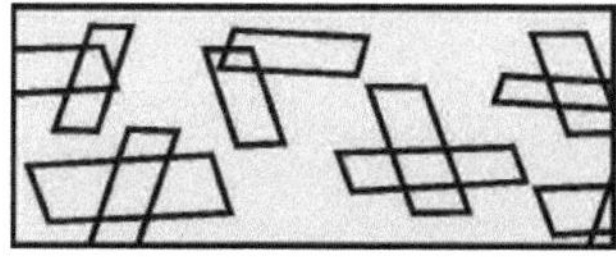

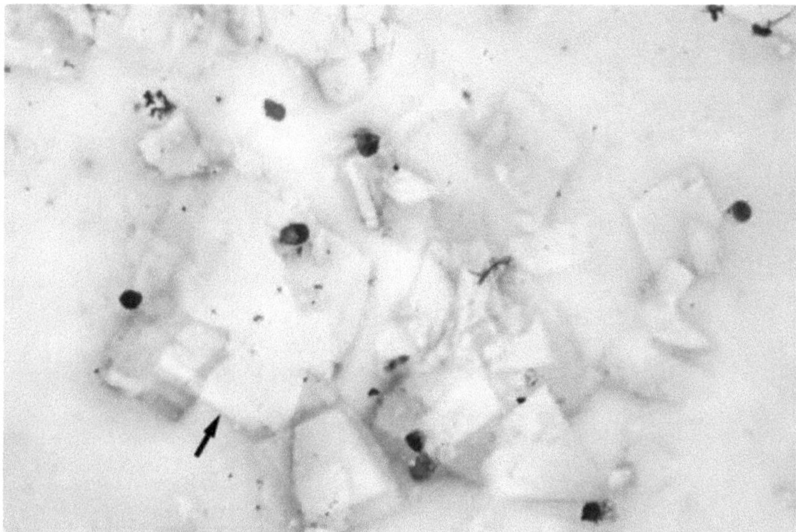

Figure 11 - Criteria used to identify cell origin and secretion products (**Maximow & Bloom, 1942; Esfoliative, 1961; Marcondes, 1975**).

Figure 11 - Breast **cholestoma** (arrow). CCA - fine needle aspiration. Bitch. GIEMSA, 40x.

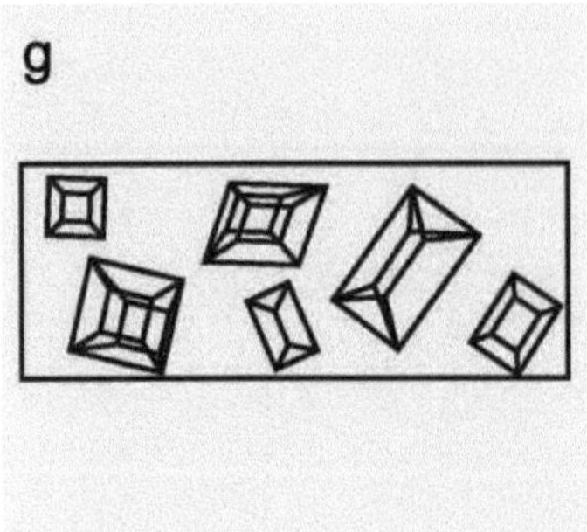

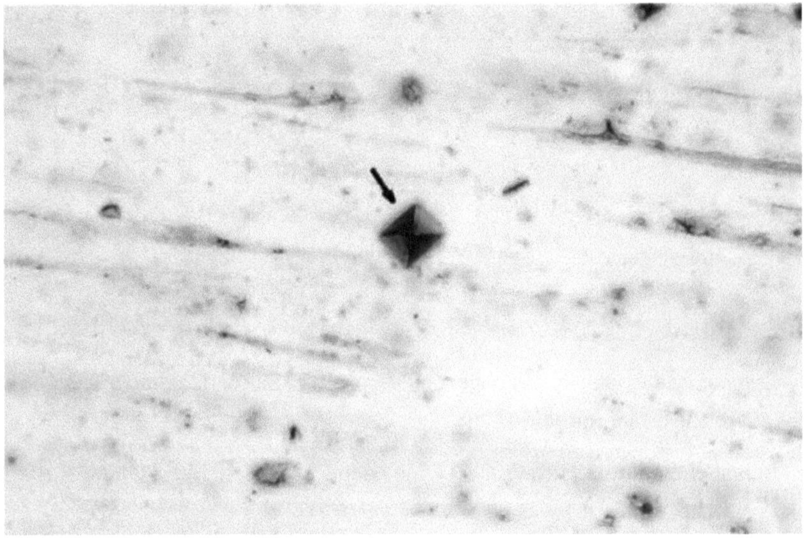

Figure 11 - Criteria used to identify cell origin and secretion products (**Maximow & Bloom, 1942; Esfoliative, 1961; Marcondes, 1975**).- Oxalate crystals.

Figura 11 - Oxalate crystal (arrow). CEE - feline bladder lavage. GIEMSA, 40x.

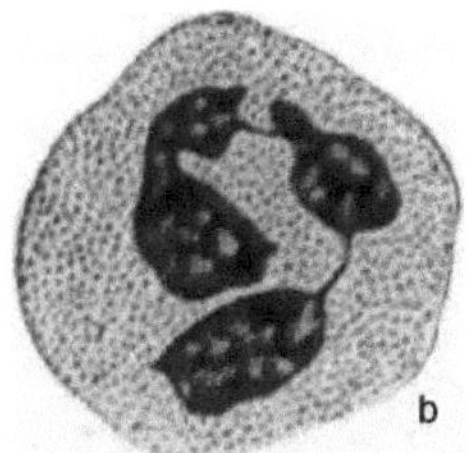

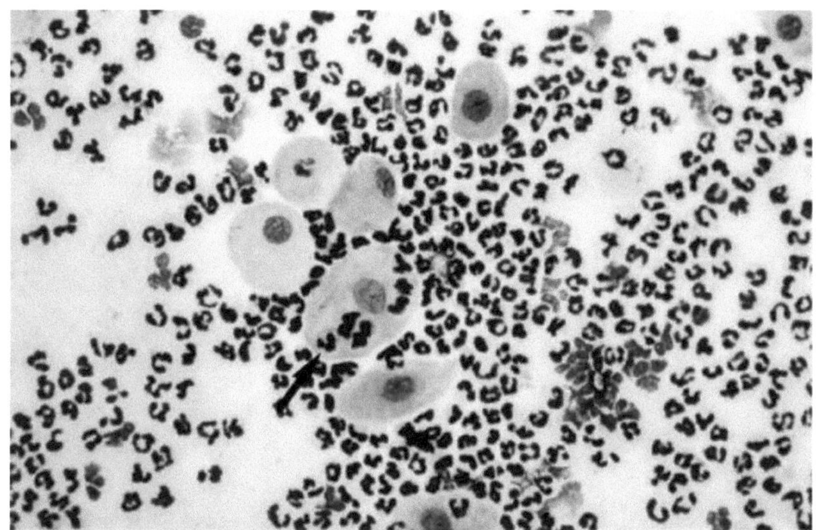

Figura 12 - Criteria for identifying the components of inflammation (**Maximow & Bloom, 1942; Esfoliative, 1961; Marcondes, 1975**). **a** - non-specific acute inflammation; **b** - neutrophil;

Figura 13 - Nonspecific conjunctivitis (arrow). CEI - impression by degenerated cellulose membrane

.

External ocular conjunctiva of cancer. GIEMSA, 20x.

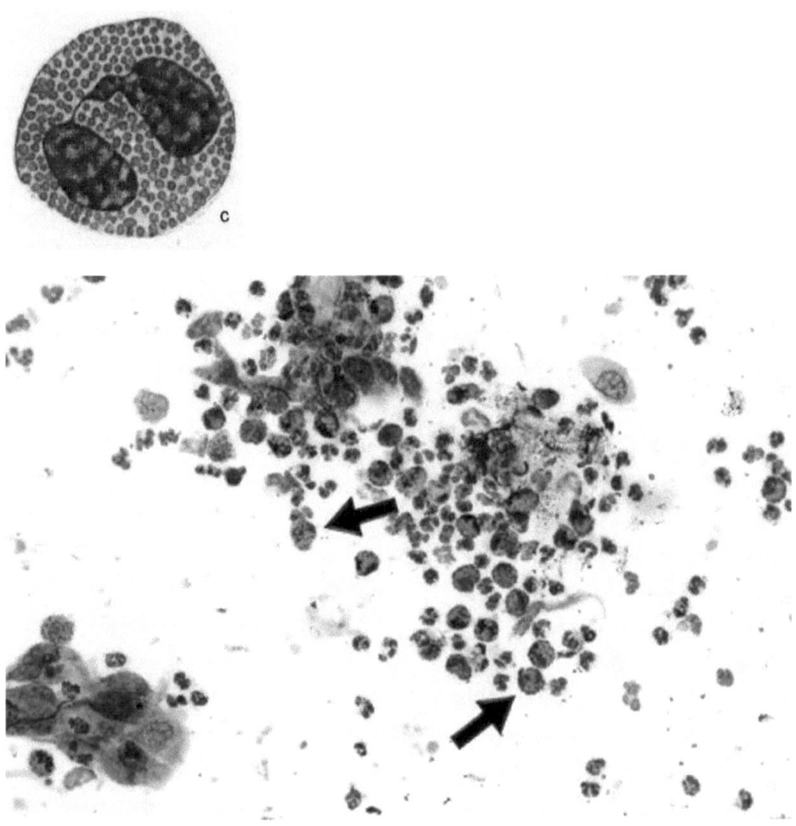

Figure 12 - Criteria for identifying the components of inflammation (**Maximow & Bloom, 1942; Esfoliative, 1961; Marcondes, 1975**).

a - nonspecific acute inflammation; **b** - neutrophil; **c** - eosinophil; **d** - plasma cell; **e** - mast cell; **f** - lymphocyte; **g** - blood cell and h - macrophage.

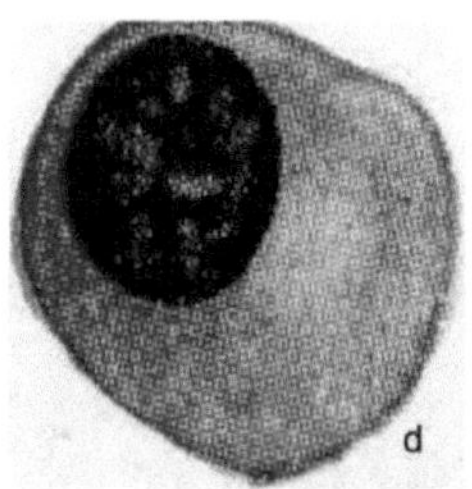

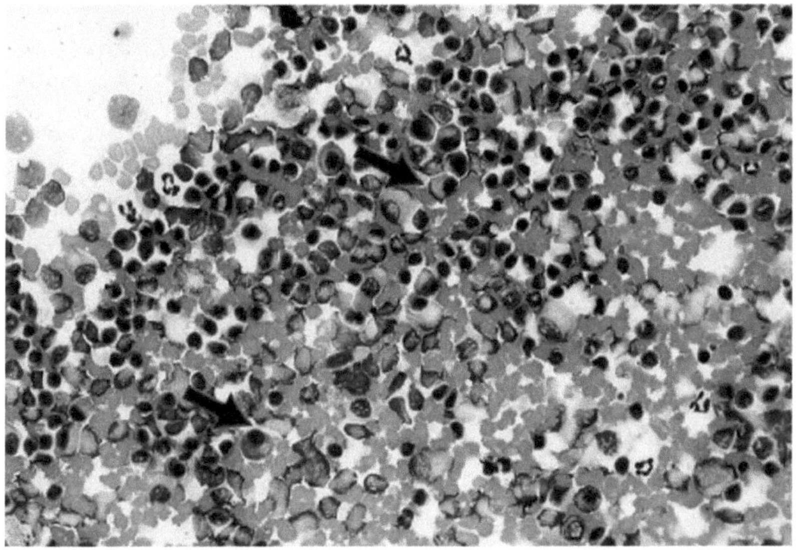

Figure 12 - Criteria for identifying the components of inflammation (**Maximow & Bloom, 1942; Esfoliative, 1961; Marcondes, 1975**).

a - nonspecific acute inflammation; **b** - neutrophil; **c** - eosinophil; **d** - plasma cell; **e** - mast cell; **f** - lymphocyte; **g** - blood cell and h - macrophage.

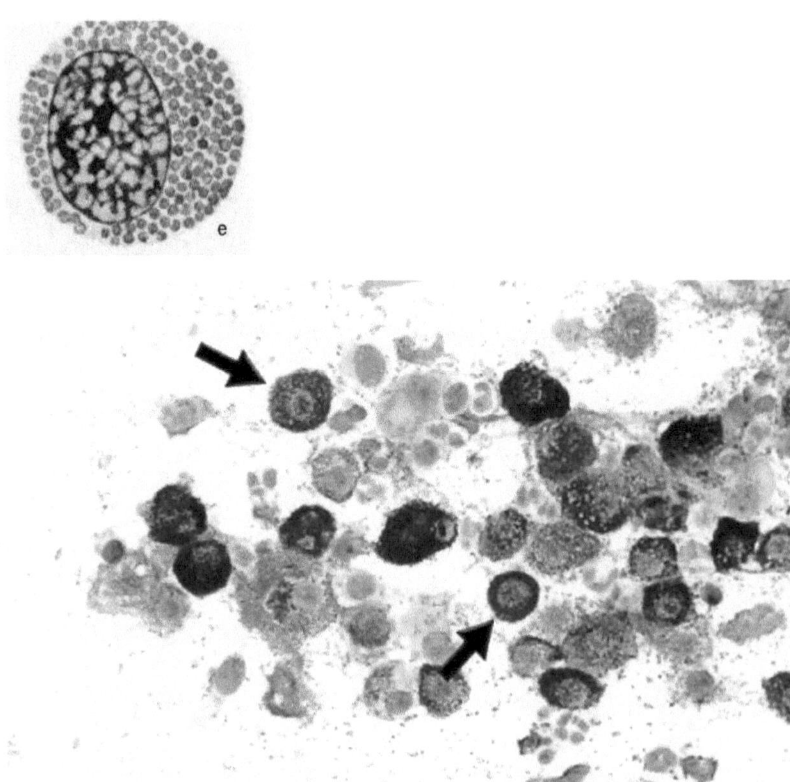

Figure 12 - Criteria for identifying the components of inflammation (**Maximow & Bloom, 1942; Esfoliative, 1961; Marcondes, 1975**).

a - nonspecific acute inflammation; **b** - neutrophil; **c** - eosinophil; **d** - plasma cell; **e** - mast cell; **f** - lymphocyte; **g** - red blood cell and h - macrophage.

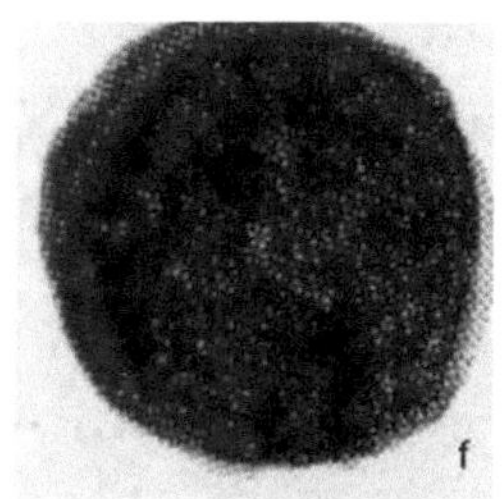

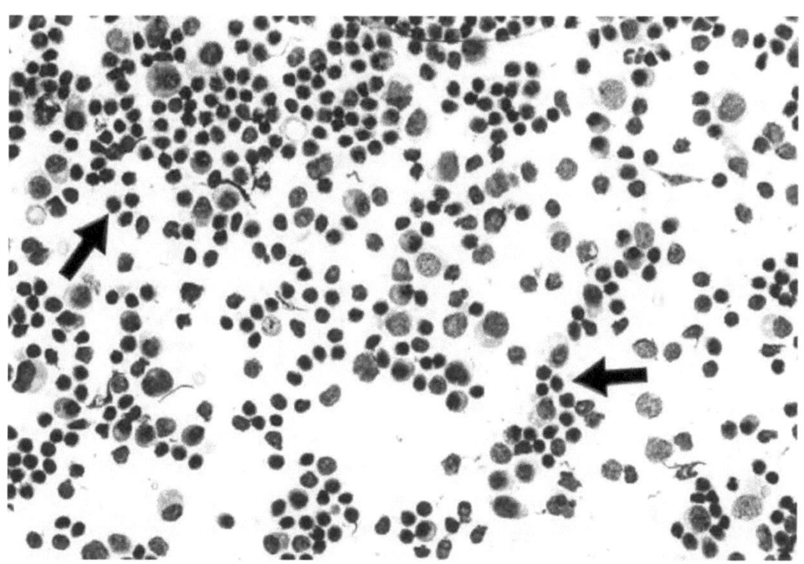

Figure 12 - Criteria for identifying the components of inflammation (**Maximow & Bloom, 1942; Esfoliative, 1961; Marcondes, 1975**).

a - nonspecific acute inflammation; **b** - neutrophil; **c** - eosinophil; **d** - plasma cell; **e** - mast cell; **f** - lymphocyte; **g** - blood cell and h - macrophage.

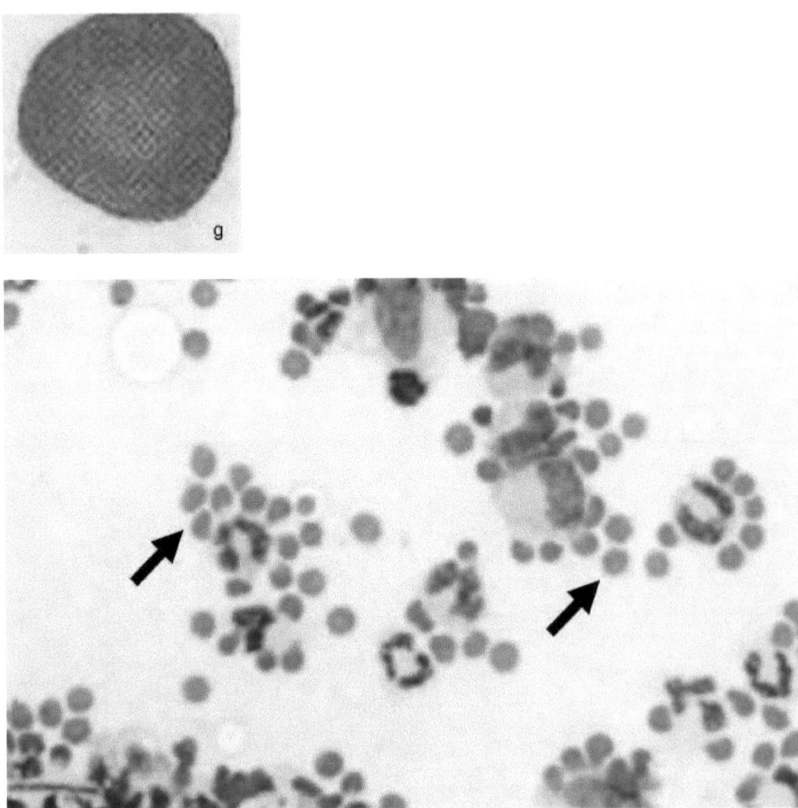

Figure 12 - Criteria for identifying the components of inflammation (**Maximow & Bloom, 1942; Esfoliative, 1961; Marcondes, 1975**).

a - nonspecific acute inflammation; **b** - neutrophil; **c** - eosinophil; **d** - plasma cell; **e** - mast cell; **f** - lymphocyte; **g** - blood cell and h - macrophage.

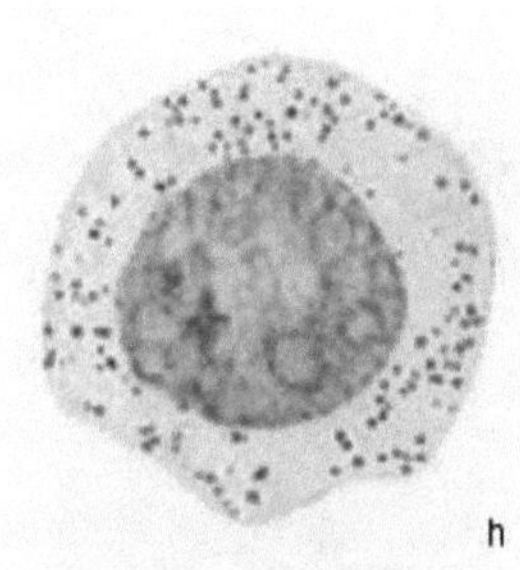

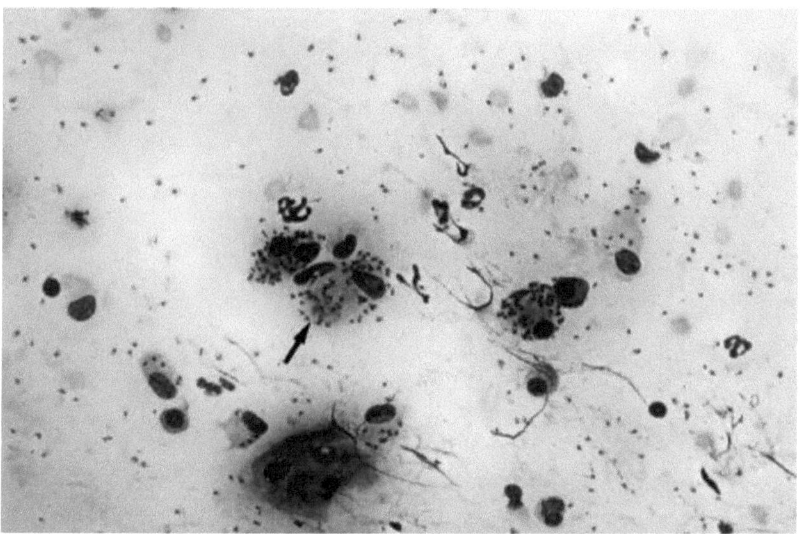

Figura 12 - Criteria for identifying the components of inflammation (**Maximow & Bloom, 1942; Esfoliative, 1961; Marcondes, 1975**).- macrophage.

Figura 13 - Cutaneous leishmaniasis (arrow). CCA - fine needle aspiration. Dog skin. GIEMSA, 20x.

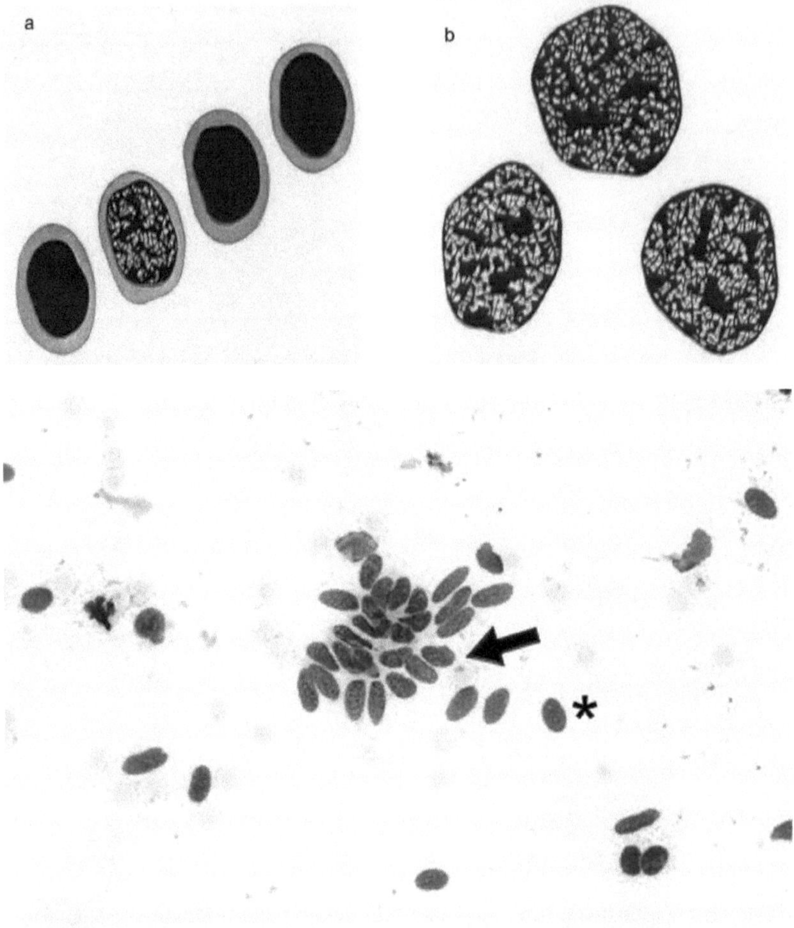

Figura 14 - Criteria used to identify the cohesive and threshed forms of cells on the histological slide (**Esfoliative, 1961; Marcondes, 1975; Acta Cytological, 1998**).

a - Cells arranged in single file; **b** - Absence of cytoplasm, irregular outline, abundant and dispersed chromatin and loss of adhesion; **c** - Cytoplasmic vacuolization, aberrant nucleolus, anisocytosis and superposition.

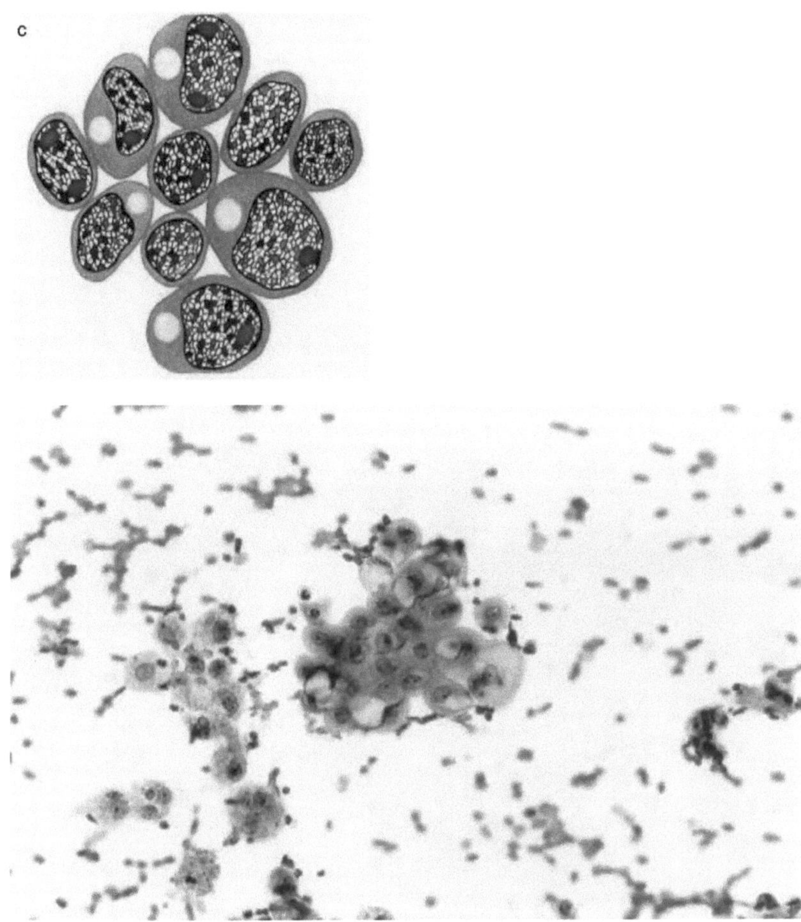

Figure 13 - Criteria used to identify the cohesive and debulked forms of cells on the histological slide (**Esfoliative, 1961; Marcondes, 1975; Acta Cytological, 1998**).

a - Cells arranged in single file; **b** - Absence of cytoplasm, irregular outline, abundant and dispersed chromatin and loss of adhesion; **c** - Cytoplasmic vacuolization, aberrant nucleolus, anisocytosis and superposition.

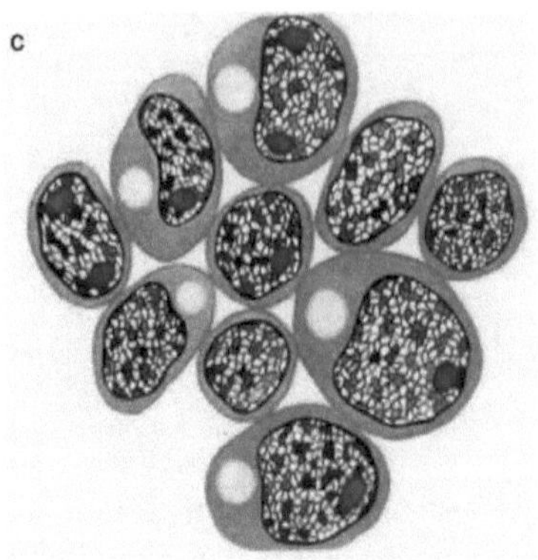

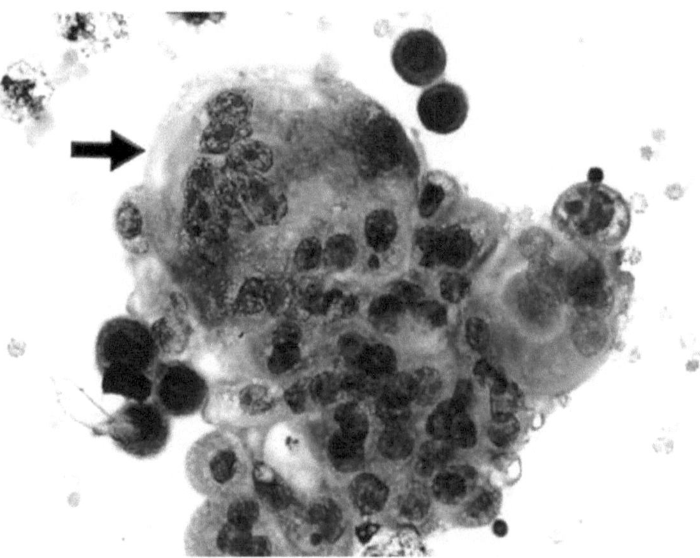

Figure 13 - Criteria used to identify the cohesive and threshed forms of cells on the histological slide (**Esfoliative, 1961; Marcondes, 1975;**

Acta Cytological, 1998).

a - Cells arranged in single file; **b** - Absence of cytoplasm, irregular outline, abundant and dispersed chromatin and loss of adhesion; **c** - Cytoplasmic vacuolization, aberrant nucleolus, anisocytosis and superposition.

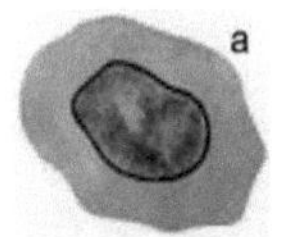
a

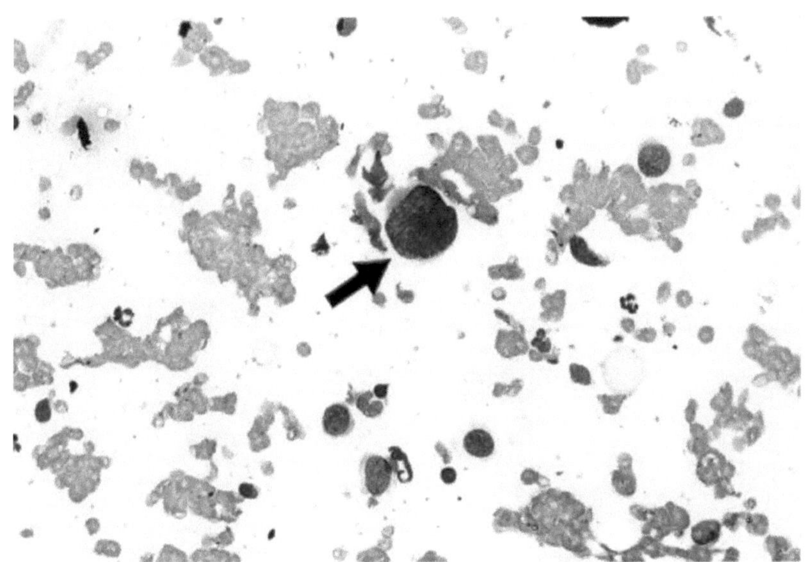

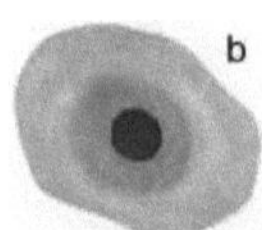
b

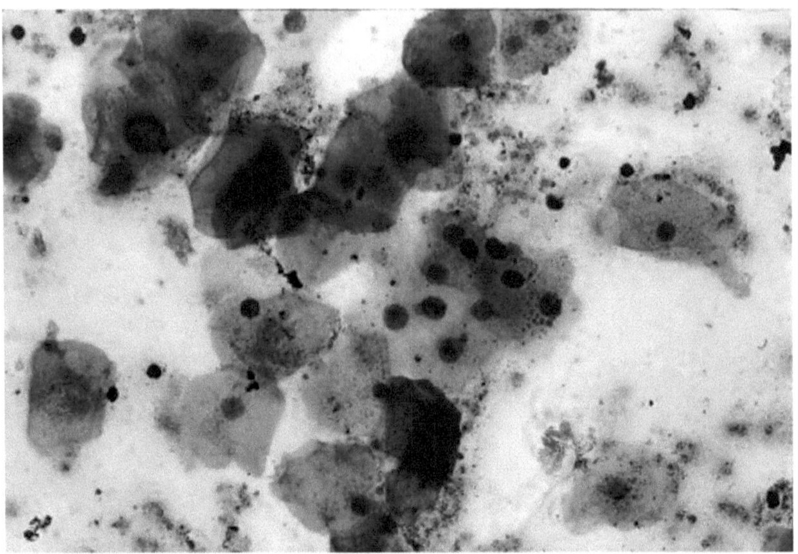

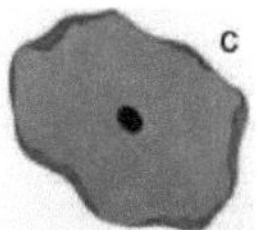

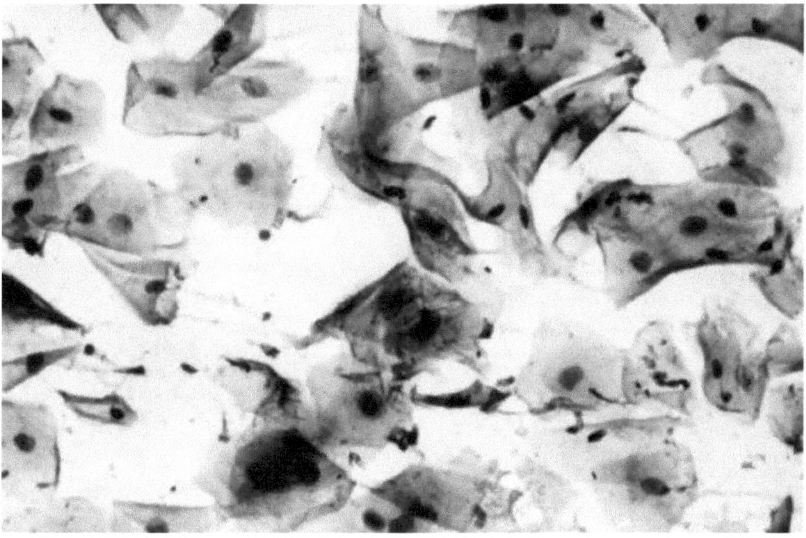

Figure 18 - Standardization of the technique and staining of the sample - CEI - AYRA spatula

AYRA. Dog gingival conjunctiva. Shorr, 40x.

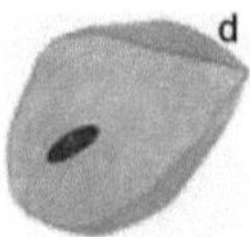

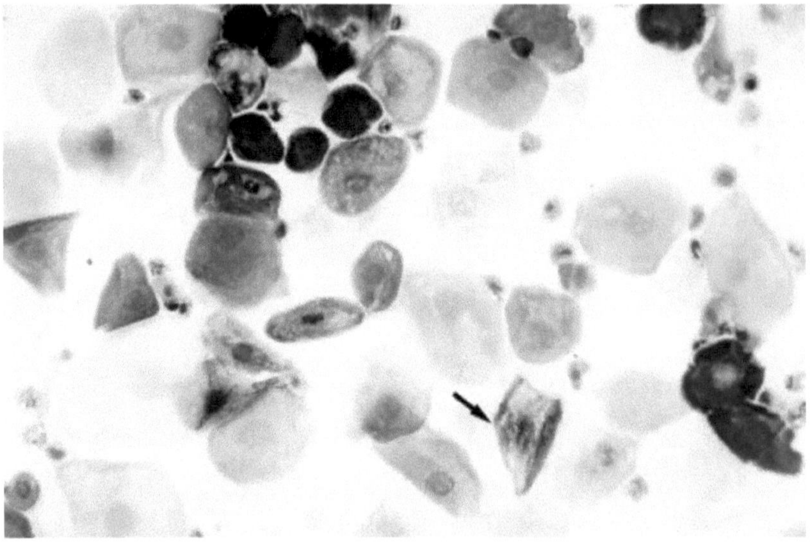

Figure 33 - Hormonal influence (arrow). CEI - Ayra's spatula. Vaginal mucosa of pregnancy. Navicular cell (arrow). Bitch. Shorr, 40x.

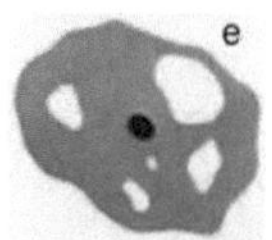
e

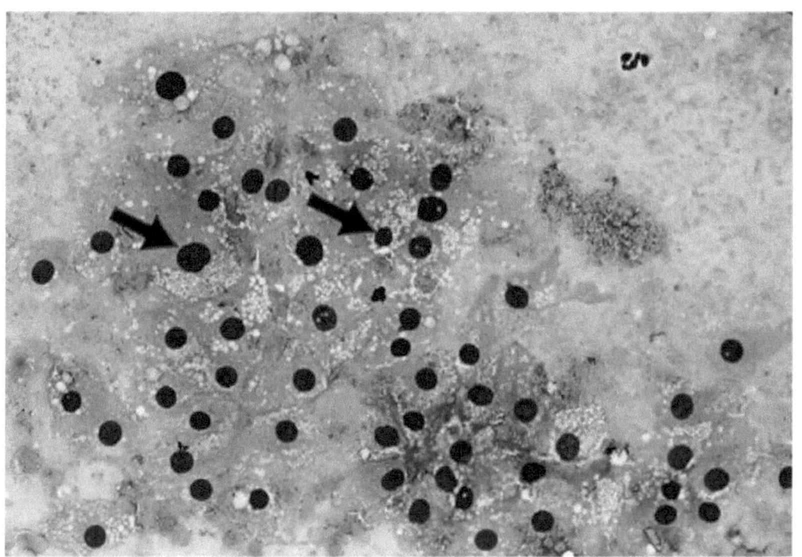

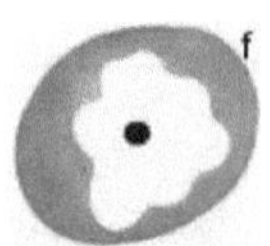
f

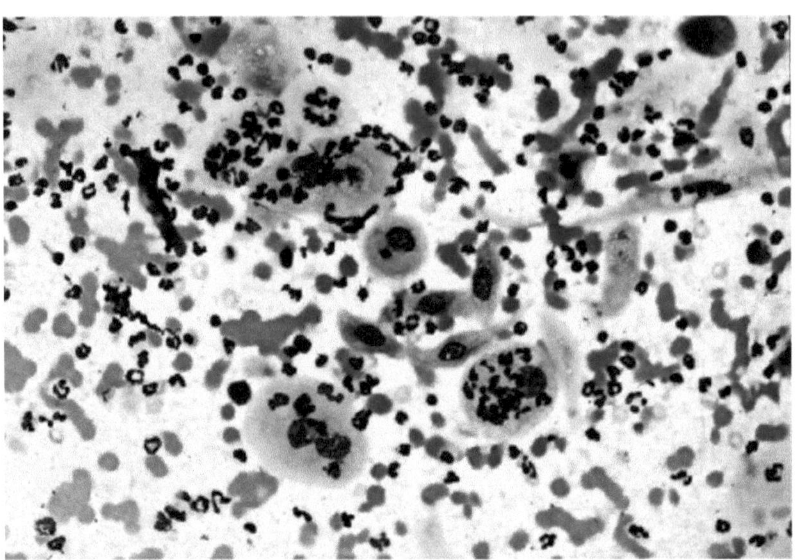

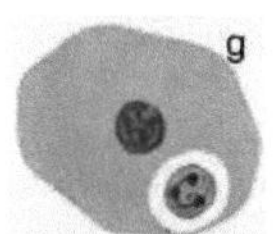
g

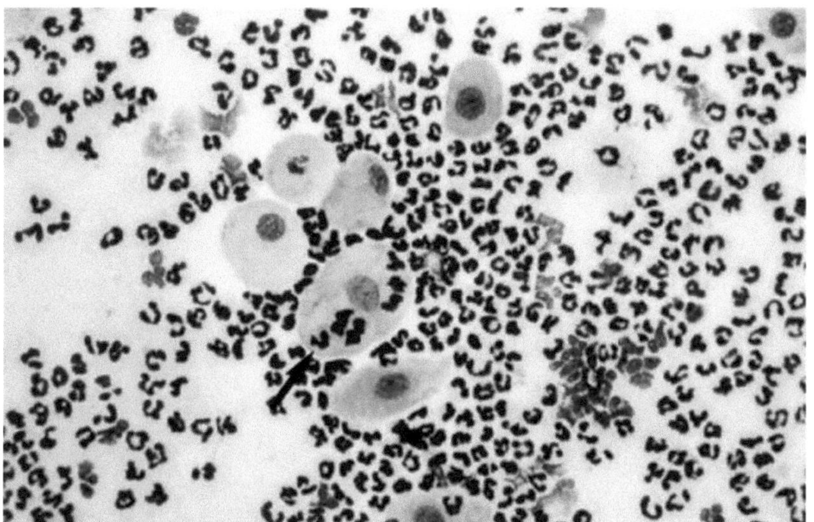

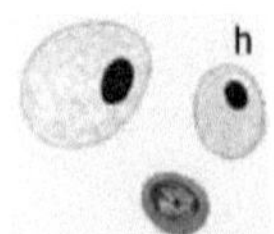
h

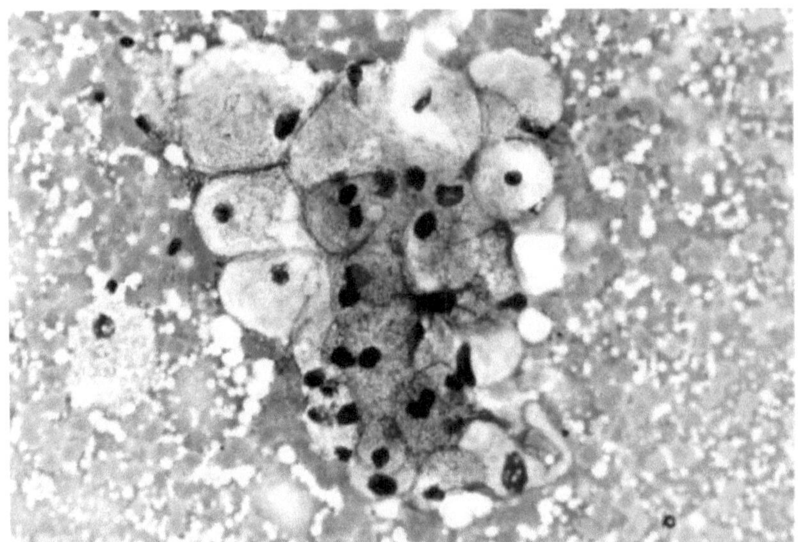

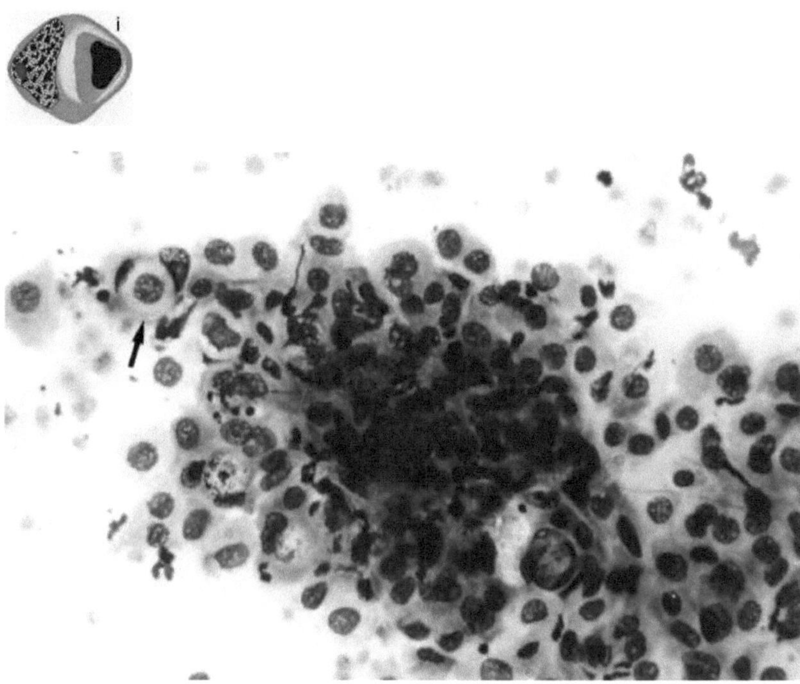

Figure 45 - Inflammatory carcinoma. Fine needle aspiration. Bitch. Cannibalism (arrow). GIEMSA, 40x.

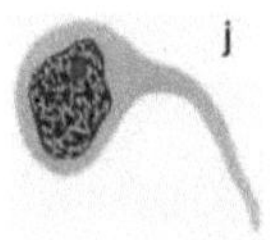
j

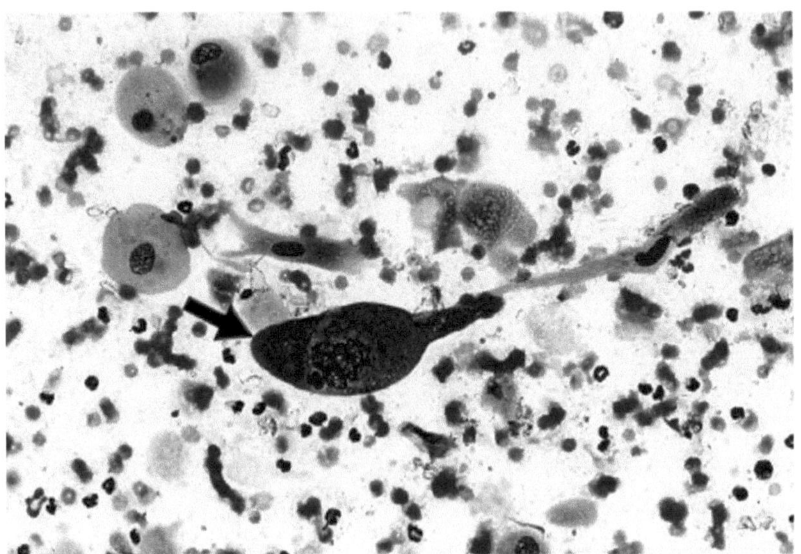

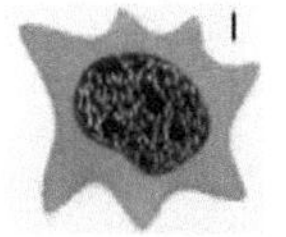

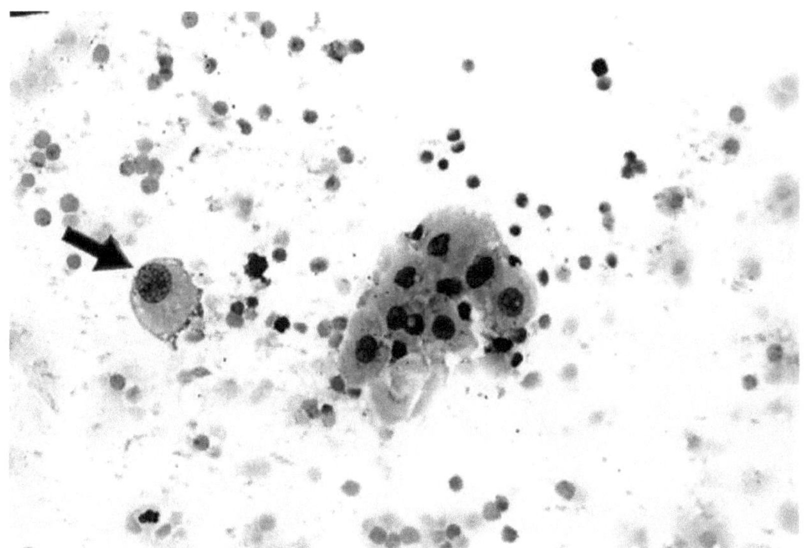

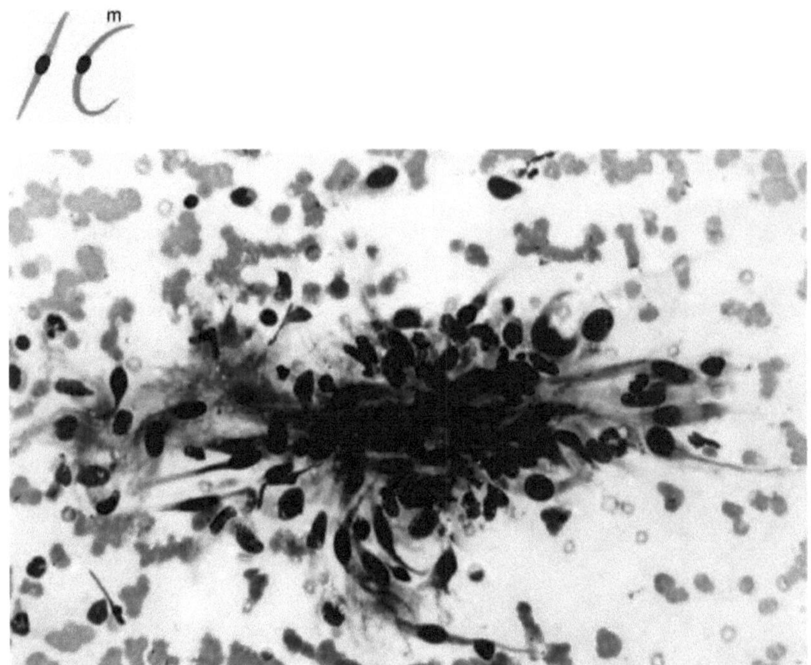

Figure 54 -Rabdomyosarcoma. CCC - fine needle aspiration. Dog. GIEMSA, 40x.

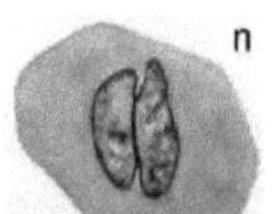
n

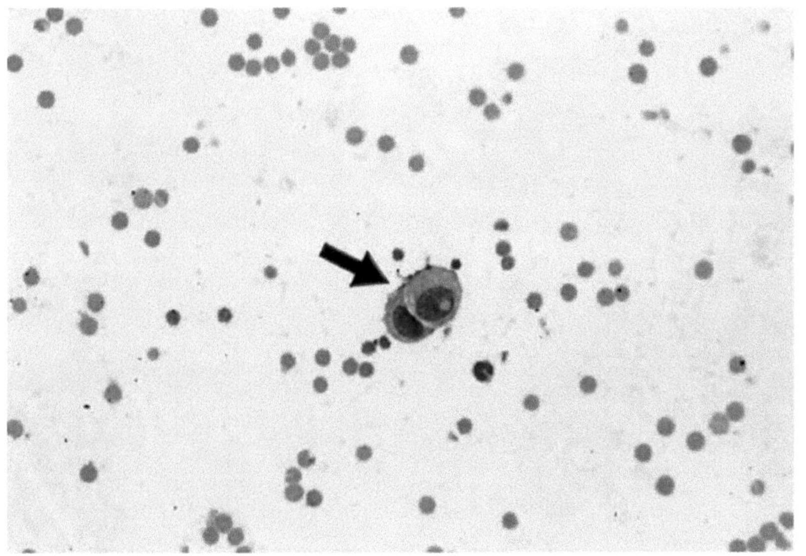

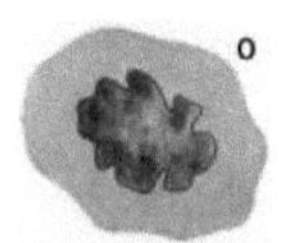

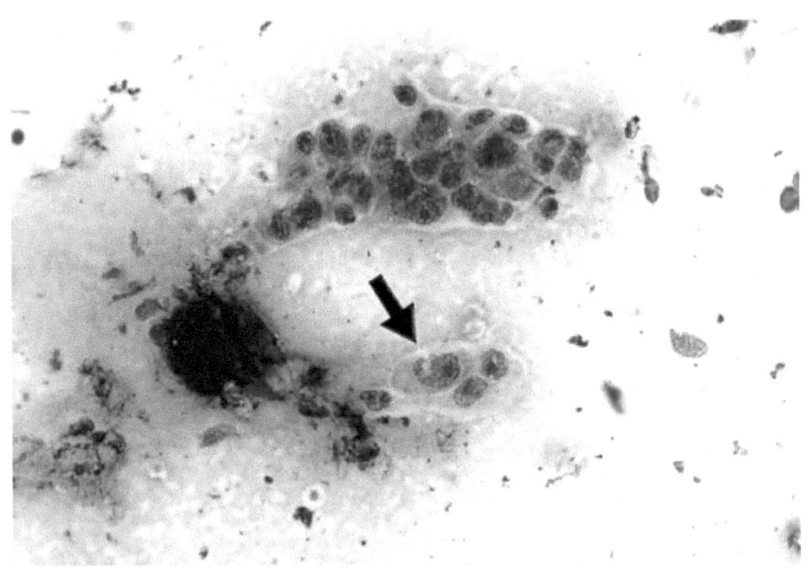

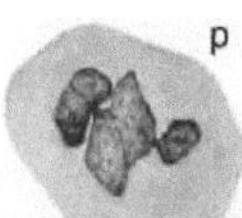

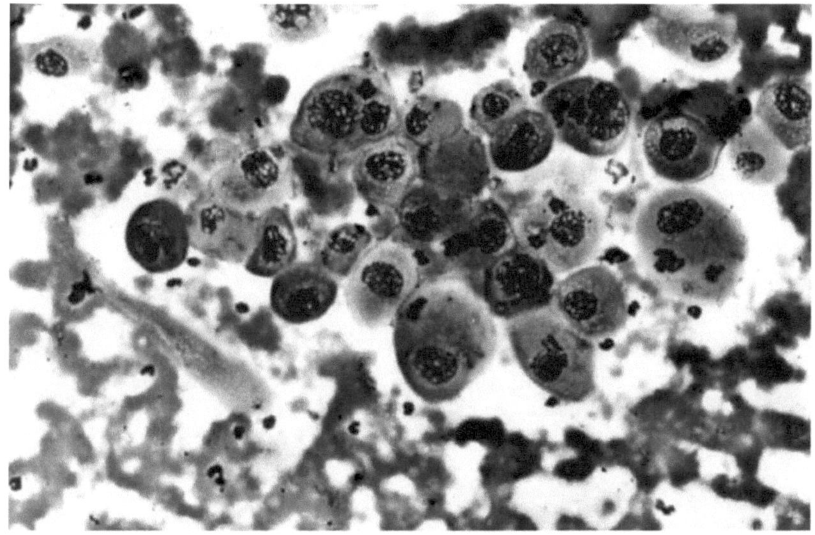

Figure 44 - Laryngeal carcinoma. CCA - fine needle aspiration. Camera. GIEMSA, 40x.

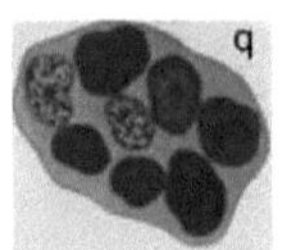

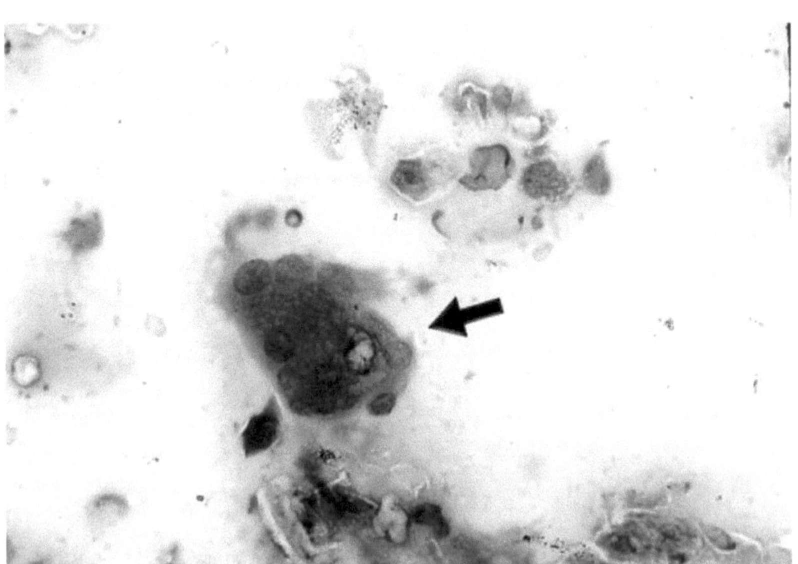

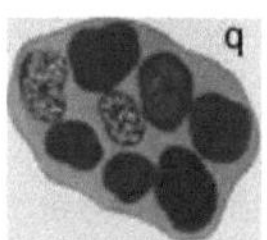

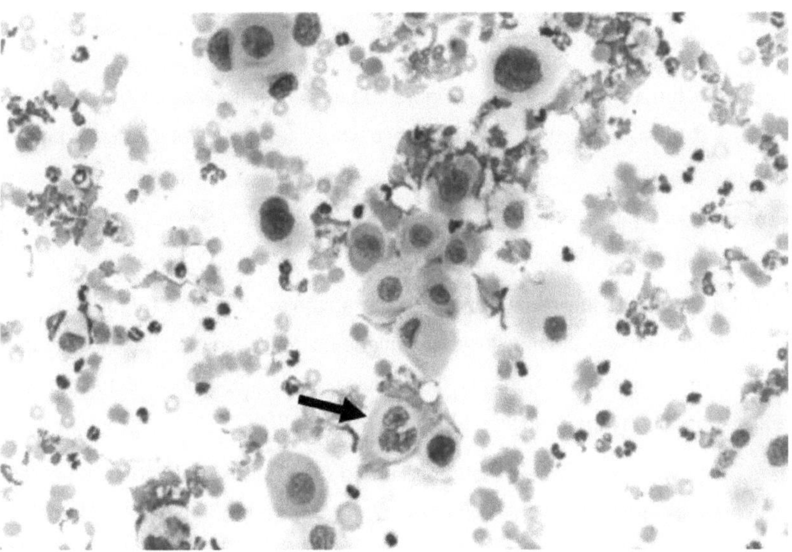

Figure 14 - Criteria for identifying tissue cells that are neoplastic and/or attacked by inflammatory injury (**Esfoliative, 1961; Marcondes, 1975; McKee, 1977; Carvalho, 1993; Acta Cytological, 1998**).

a - Hyperchromatic nuclear membrane: caries, inflammation and neoplasia; **b** - Metachromasia: inflammation; **c and d** - Cytoplasmic folding: inflammation and progesterone; **e to i** - Cytoplasmic vacuolization: repair, phagocytosis, dysplasia and cannibalism (when the phagocytosed cell is of the same origin as the one that phagocytosed it); **j, l and m** - Tadpole cell, or racket, amoebic and fiber: malignancy **and n and o** - nuclear molding and irregular nuclear contour: degeneration, viral infection, malignancy and micro-invasion **and p and q** - multinucleation: inflammation, malignancy and radiation.

5. Results

During the eight years of the study, no complications were reported in the animals related to the sample collection technique, since the course of action was always decided on the basis of clinical and imaging findings (Figures 15 and 16).

With the exception of the animals in group 3 (Figures 5d and e), tranquilizers were only used on those that were extremely aggressive and/or those whose lesions were located in places that were difficult to handle.

From March 23, 1994 to July 11, 2002, the aspiration technique (CCA) (Figure 7) was the most commonly used technique for sampling lesions from animals in Groups 1 and 3 (Figures 5c, d and e). During the same period, for the animals in Group 2 (Figures 5a and b), the gynecological brush was the most used technique for collecting material. At the same time, for the animals in Group 4 (Figure 5f), the effusion sample collection technique was used more often than the lavage collection technique (Figure 6f).

In all the years, dogs were the animals that represented more groups than felines, horses, ruminants, wild animals and birds. With regard to sex, there was a predominance of females, both in the case of dogs and the other species. In terms of age group, animals aged between 6 and 10 prevailed, as can be seen in Tables 3 to 20.

5.1 Casuistry and Sample Quality for Diagnostic Cytological Examination - 1994 to 2002

During the period from March 23, 1994 to July 11, 2002, 93,939 animals of different species were treated at the UNESP Botucatu Veterinary Hospital with various clinical suspicions. Of this total, 5.27% (4,953) were submitted to cytological examination, Tables 1 and 2 and Graph 1.

Table 1 - Casuistry - Veterinary Hospital, 1994 to 2001.

Year	Number of cases attended
1994	11034
1995	11157
1996	11161
1997	12221
1998	12075
1999	11163
2000	12017
2001	13111
Total	93939

The annual evolution of cytological examinations from 1994 to 2001, as well as the diagnoses issued by the Pathology Service of the Veterinary Hospital - UNESP, are shown in Table 3.

Table 2 - Annual evolution of cytological and diagnostic tests - Veterinary Hospital, 1994 to 2002.

Cytological examination		**Diagnosis (%)**			
Year	**№/animal**	**Inflammatory**	**Non-inflammatory**	**Inconclusive***	**Insufficient**
1994	126	43 (34,13)	54 (42,86)	14 (11,11)	15 (11,90)
1995	338	125 (36,98)	166 (49,11)	16 (4,74)	31 (9,17)
1996	350	152 (43,43)	181 (51,72)	1 (0,285)	16 (4,57)
1997	448	159 (32,58)	315 (64,55)	2 (0,41)	12 (2,46)
1998	787	234 (29,73)	502 (63,79)	31 (3,94)	20 (2,54)
1999	773	330 (42,69)	426 (55,11)	6 (0,78)	11 (1,42)
2000	786	301 (38,29)	462 (58,79)	17 (2,16)	6 (0,76)
2001	876	413 (47,15)	447 (51,02)	0 (0)	16 (1,83)
2002	469	354 (75,48)	106 (22,60)	0 (0)	9 (1,92)
Total	4953	2111 (42,40)	2659 (53,40)	87 (1,60)	136 (2,60)

* Inconclusive: satisfactory but limited.

Graphs 1 and 2 show the annual evolution of the incidence of diagnoses: quantity and quality - Veterinary Hospital, 1994 to 2002.

Graph 1 - Annual evolution of samples: quantity and quality - Veterinary Hospital, 1994 to 2002.

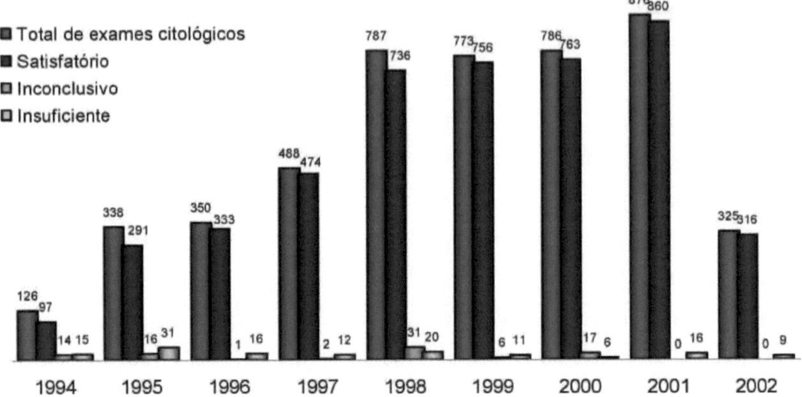

Graph 2 - Annual evolution of diagnoses: inflammation, non-inflammation, inconclusive and insufficient - Veterinary Hospital, 1994 to 2002.

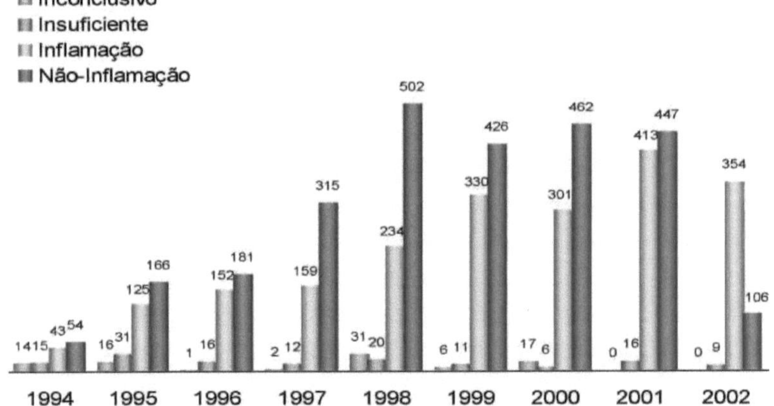

5.2 Cytological examination with diagnosis of inflammation

Diagnoses were made on the basis of clinical findings, concentration and discipline in reading the samples. Regardless of the technique used to collect the sample for cytological examination, it was possible to identify all the categories of inflammation in the animals (Figures 19 to 31). It was present in all species, sexes and age groups (Tables 3 to 20). In addition, in certain samples it was possible to identify the agent responsible for the condition (Figures 19 to 26).

5.3 Cytological Examination with Non-Inflammatory Diagnosis

The way the material was collected did not interfere, even though different equipment was used to collect cytological samples to diagnose inflammatory and non-inflammatory lesions (Figures 19 to 58).

Throughout the evaluation period, it was possible to observe cell morphology characteristic of the degenerative, dysplastic, hyperplastic (Figures 34 to 36) and neoplastic processes. In the latter, it was possible to classify them as epithelial, mesenchymal and round cell (Figures 41 to 58).

Among the neoplasms, the most significant was breast cancer in bitches, followed by transmissible venereal tumor, lymphoma and mastocytoma in dogs (Figures 43, 46, 48, 49 and 53). It was also possible to identify the morphology of lesions not yet described in veterinary cytopathology literature (Figures 32).

Table 3 - Incidence of inflammatory and non-inflammatory lesions: male and female dogs - Veterinary Hospital, 1994.

Age group	**Inflammation**		**No - inflammation**	
	%	&	%	&
0-5	11	3	7	2
6-10	2	4	12	19
11-15		1	4	5
16-20			1	
Total	13	8	24	26

Table 4 - Incidence of inflammatory and non-inflammatory lesions: male and female cats, cattle and horses - Veterinary Hospital, 1994.

Age group	**Inflammation**		**No - inflammation**	
	%	&	%	&
0-5	1	2		3
6-10				
11-15		1	1	
16-20				
Total	1	3	1	3

Table 5 - Incidence of inflammatory and non-inflammatory lesions: male and female dogs - Veterinary Hospital, 1995.

Age group		Inflammation	No inflammation	
%		&	%	&
0-59		8	25	27
6-1013		15	44	35
11-153		10	4	27
16-20	-			2
Total	25	33	73	91

Table 6 - Incidence of inflammatory and non-inflammatory lesions: felines and bovines, males and females - Veterinary Hospital, 1995.

Age group	Inflammation		No - inflammation	
	%	&	%	&
0-5		1		
6-10	1	1		2
И ИС				
11-15				
16-20				
Total	1	2	0	2

Table 7 - Incidence of inflammatory and non-inflammatory lesions: male and female dogs - Veterinary Hospital, 1996.

Age group	Inflammation		No - inflammation	
	%	&	%	&
0-5	28	16	17	28
6-10	20	17	31	52
11-15	5	3	14	28
16-20				4
Total	53	36	62	112

Table 8 - Incidence of inflammatory and non-inflammatory lesions: male and female cats and horses - Veterinary Hospital, 1996.

Age group	Inflammation		No - inflammation	
	%	&	%	&
0-5				
6-10			1	
11-15				3
16-20				
Total	0	0	1	3

Table 9 - Incidence of inflammatory and non-inflammatory lesions: male and female dogs - Veterinary Hospital, 1997.

Age group	Inflammation		Non-inflammation	
	%	&	%	&
0-5	43	20	55	50
6-10	22	16	45	101
11-15	6	3	14	32
16-20				3
Total	61	39	104	110

Table 10 - Incidence of inflammatory and non-inflammatory lesions: male and female cats, cattle and horses - Veterinary Hospital, 1997.

Age group	Inflammation		No - inflammation	
	%	&	%	&
0-5	4	2	2	2
6-10			1	5
11-15		1		4
16-20				
Total	4	3	3	11

Table 11 - Incidence of inflammatory and non-inflammatory lesions: male and female dogs - Veterinary Hospital, 1998.

Age group	Inflammation		No - inflammation	
	%	&	%	&
0-5	42	28	85	78
6-10	29	33	75	153
11-15	9	11	31	49
16-20			1	7
Total	60	72	182	287

Table 12 - Incidence of inflammatory and non-inflammatory lesions: felines, ruminants, birds and wild animals, males and females - Veterinary Hospital, 1998.

Age group	Inflammation		No inflammation	
	%	&	%	&
0-5	-	6	1	2
6-10		4	1	6
11-15		1		3
16-20				1
Total	0	11	2	12

Table 13 - Incidence of inflammatory and non-inflammatory lesions: male and female dogs - Veterinary Hospital, 1999.

Age group	Inflammation		Non-inflammation	
	%	&	%	&
0-5	54	32	59	54
6-10	63	44	72	142
11-15	20	22	22	49
16-20		1	2	4
Total	137	99	155	429

Table 14 - Incidence of inflammatory and non-inflammatory lesions: male and female felines, horses, birds and wild animals - Veterinary Hospital, 1999.

Age group	**Inflammation**		**No inflammation**	
	%	&	%	&
0-5	5	5	2	
6-10	1	3	1	7
11-15			4	
16-20			- 1	
Total	6	8	1	14

Table 15 - Incidence of inflammatory and non-inflammatory lesions: male and female dogs - Veterinary Hospital, 2000.

Age group	**Inflammation**		**Non-inflammation**	
	%	&	%	&
0-5	47	46	62	58
6-10	55	62	87	128
11-15	16	14	36	45
16-20	2	14	1	65
Total	120	136	186	296

Table 16 - Incidence of inflammatory and non-inflammatory lesions: felines, bovines, equines, birds and wild animals, males and females - Veterinary Hospital, 2000.

	Inflammation		**Non-inflammation**	
Age group	%	&	%	&
0-5	7	6	1	2
6-10	3	3	3	9
11-15			3	
16-20				1
Total	10	9	7	12

Table 17 - Incidence of inflammatory and non-inflammatory lesions: male and female dogs - Veterinary Hospital, 2001.

Age group	**Inflammation**		**Non-inflammation**	
	%	&	%	&
0-5	47	46	62	58
6-10	55	62	87	128
11-15	16	14	36	45
16-20	2	14	1	65
Total	120	136	186	296

Table 18 - Incidence of inflammatory and non-inflammatory lesions: felines, ruminants and birds, males and females - Veterinary Hospital, 2001.

	Inflammation		**Non-inflammation**	
Age group	%	&	%	&
0-5	6	7	4	4
6-10	1	1	3	4
11-15				6
16-20				4
Total	7	8	7	18

Table 19 - Incidence of inflammatory and non-inflammatory lesions: male and female dogs - Veterinary Hospital, 2002.

Age group	**Inflammation**		**No inflammation**	
	%	&	%	&
0-5	14	22	49	52
6-10	14	28	68	94
11-15	4	7	21	38
16-20	2	1	-	-
Total	34	58	138	184

Table 20 - Incidence of inflammatory and non-inflammatory lesions: felines, ruminants, equines, wild birds, males and females - Veterinary Hospital, 2002.

Age group	Inflammation		No - inflammation	
	%	&	%	&
0-5	10	3	6	2
6-10	3	-	-3	
11-15	1	-	-2	
16-20	-	1	-1	
Total	14	4	6	8

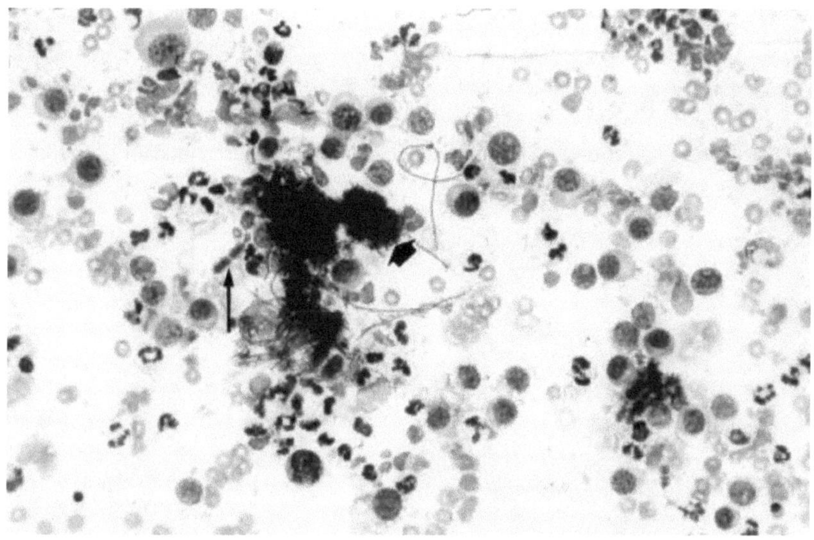

Figura 19 - Transmissible venereal tumor associated with bacterial globia (short arrow), *simonsiella* sp (long arrow) - CEI - gynecological brush. Dog nasal sinus. GIEMSA, 20x.

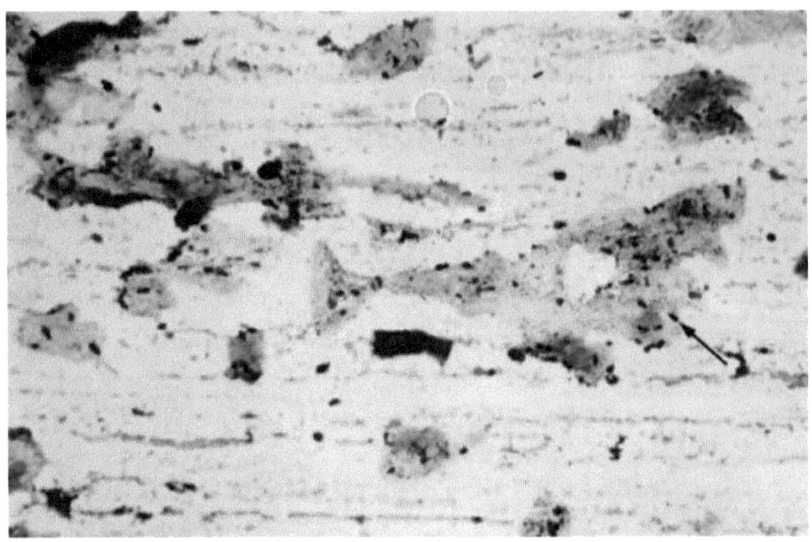

Figura 20 - *Malassezia* sp (arrow) - CEI - gynecological brush. External auditory canal of a dog. GIEMSA, 20x.

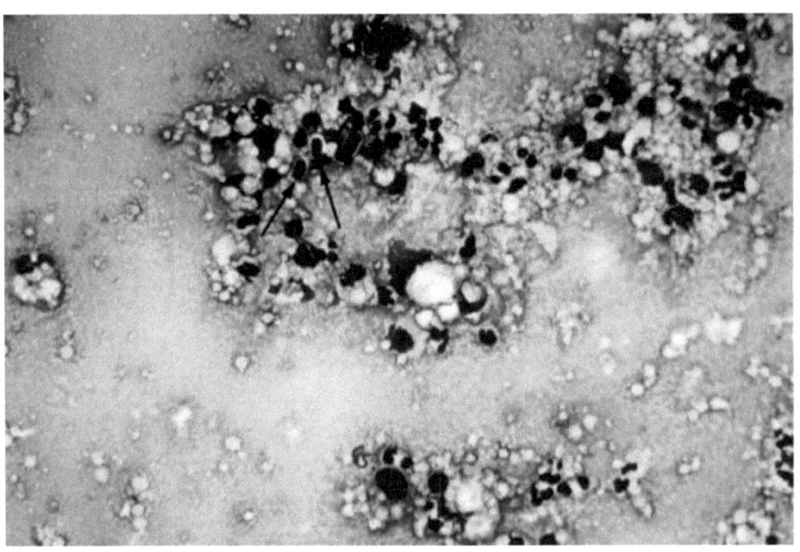

Figura 21 - Specific mastitis - *Prototeca* sp (arrows). CCA - fine needle aspiration. Goat's breast. GIEMSA, 20x.

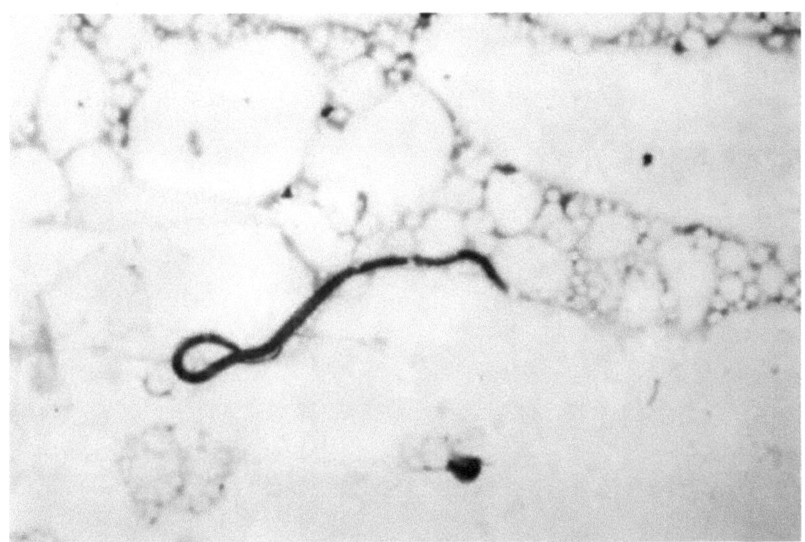

Figura 22 - Microfilaria. CCA - fine needle aspiration. Dog skin. GIEMSA, 20x.

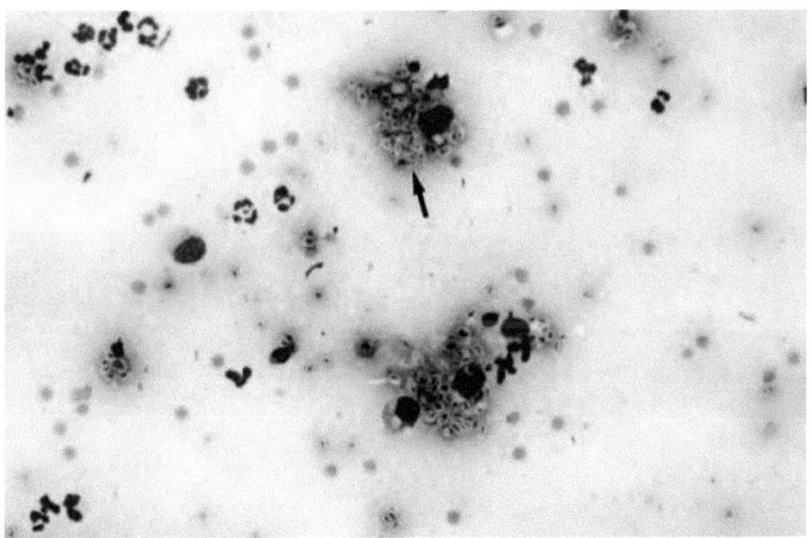

Figura 24 - Cutaneous sporotrichosis (arrow). CCA - fine needle aspiration. Feline skin. GIEMSA, 20x.

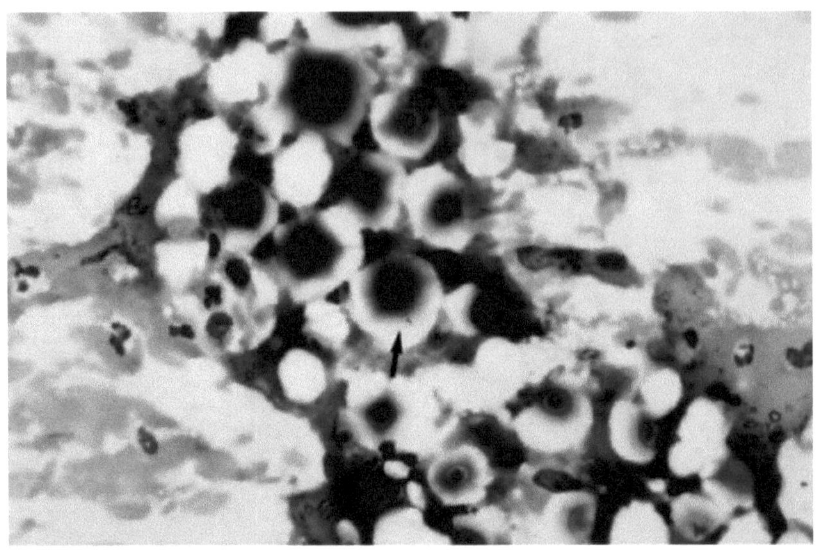

Figura 25 - Cutaneous cryptococcosis (arrow). CCA - fine needle aspiration. Dog skin. GIEMSA, 40x.

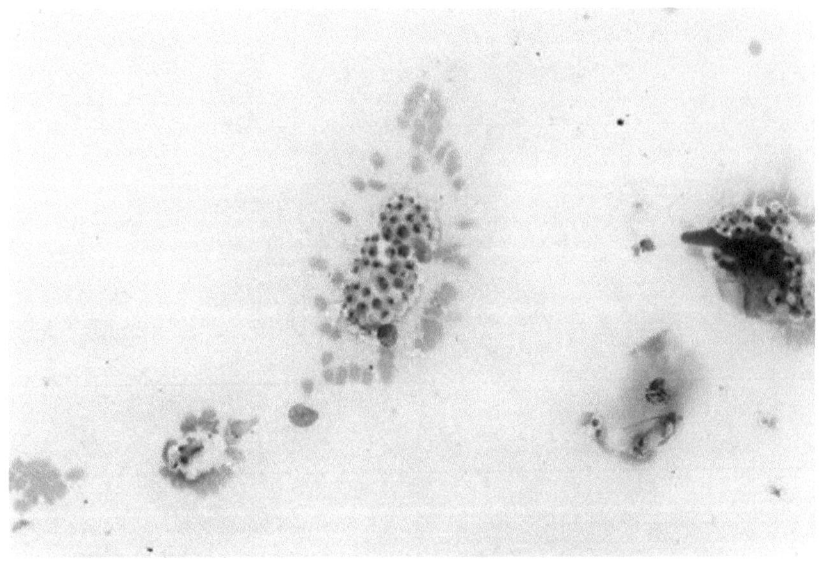

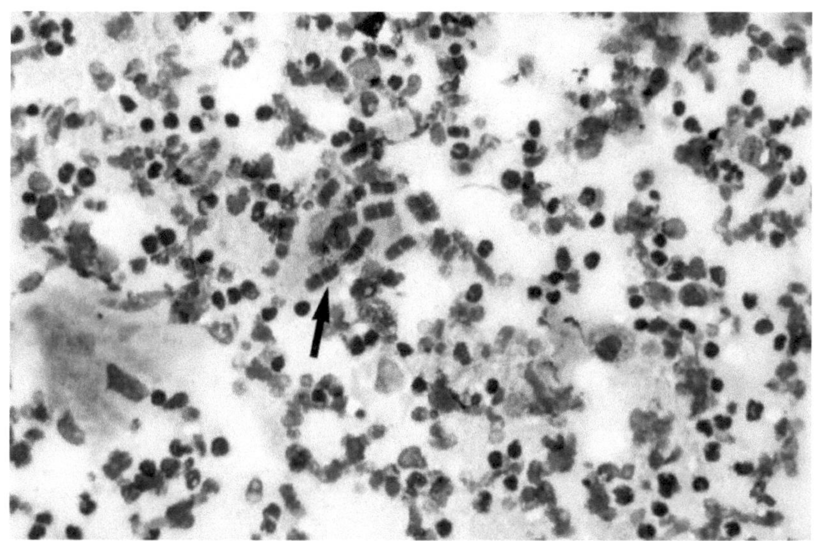

Figura 26 - Chronic pneumonia and Simonsiella sp (arrow). CEE - Tracheobronchial lavage. Dog. GIEMSA, 20x.

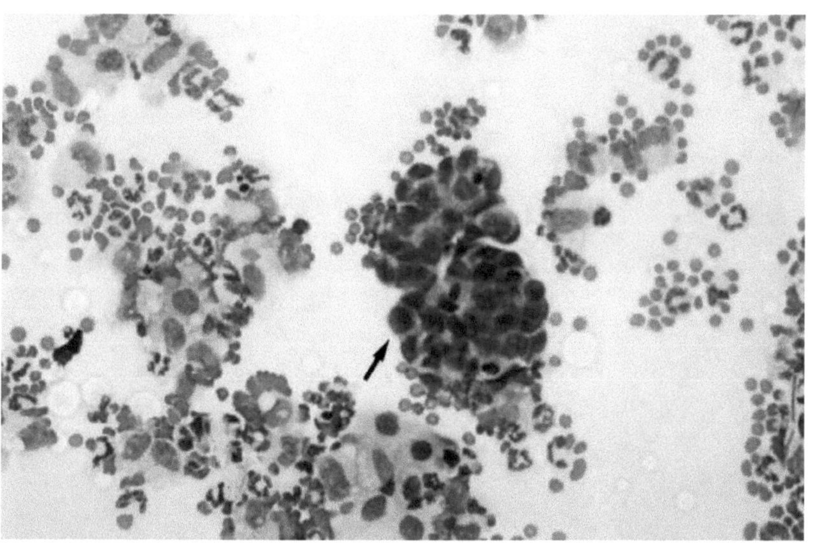

Figura 27 - Peritonitis and block of neoplastic cells (arrow). CEE - peritoneal serous effusion. Dog. GIEMSA, 20x.

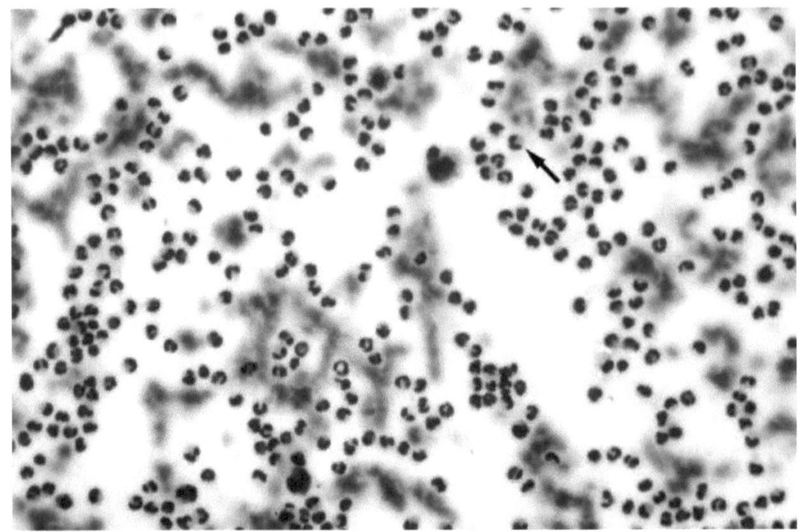

Figure 29 - Nonspecific eosinophilic folliculitis (arrow). CCA - fine needle aspiration puncture. Dog skin. GIEMSA, 20x.

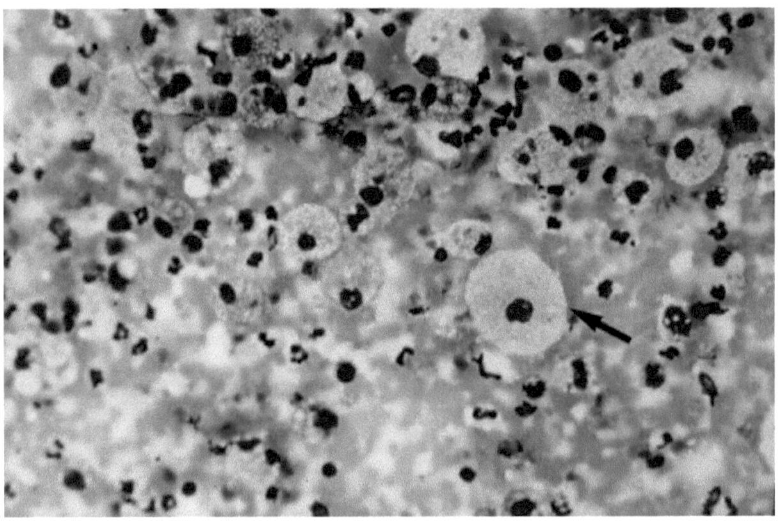

Figure 30 - Chronic mastitis (arrow). CEI - expression. Breast of dog. GIEMSA, 40x.

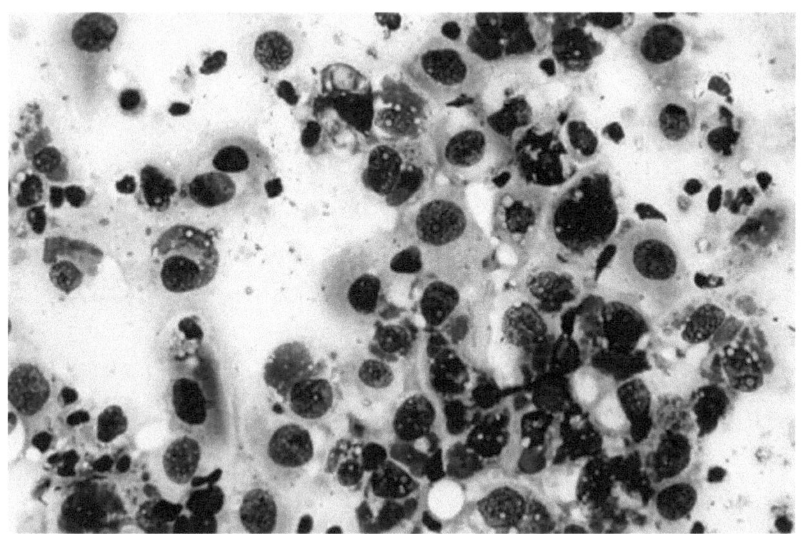

Figure 31 - Nonspecific chronic cystitis. CEE - dog bladder lavage. GIEMSA, 40x.

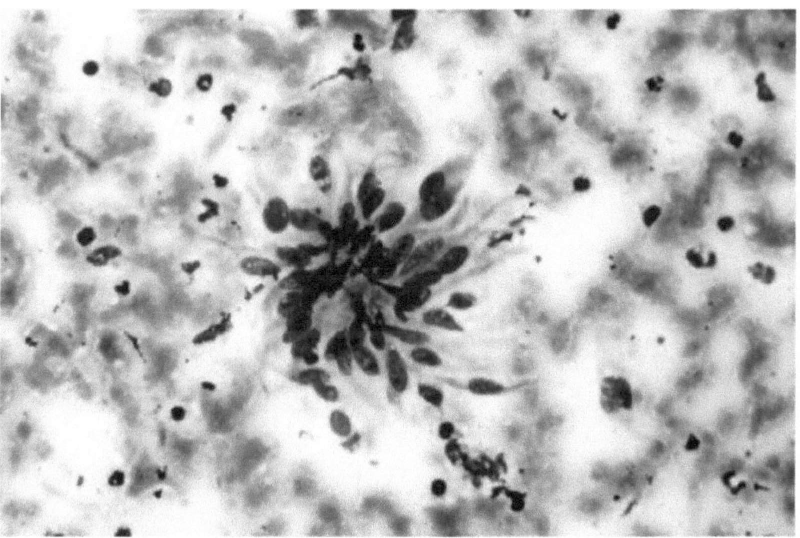

Figure 32 - Pseudo inflammatory tumor - CCA - fine needle aspiration. Cancer bladder. GIEMSA, 20x.

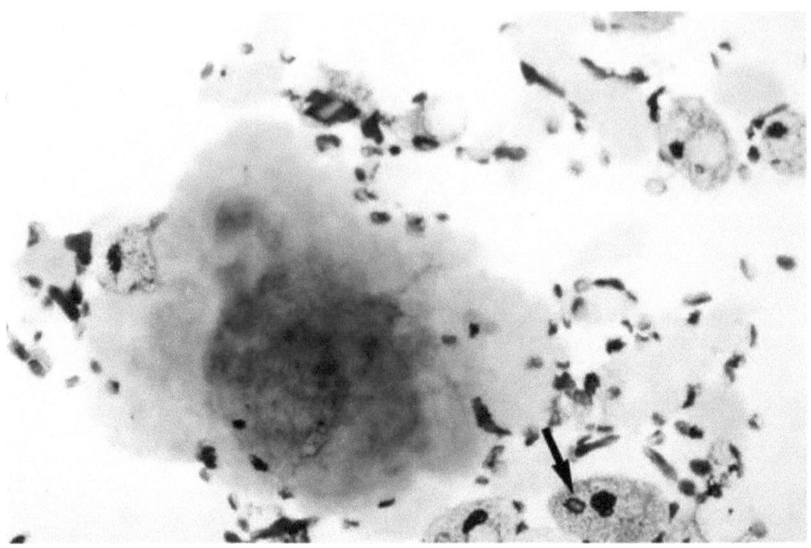

Figure 34 - Mucocele. CCA - fine needle aspiration, salivary gland of cancer. Crystals (arrow). GIEMSA, 40x.

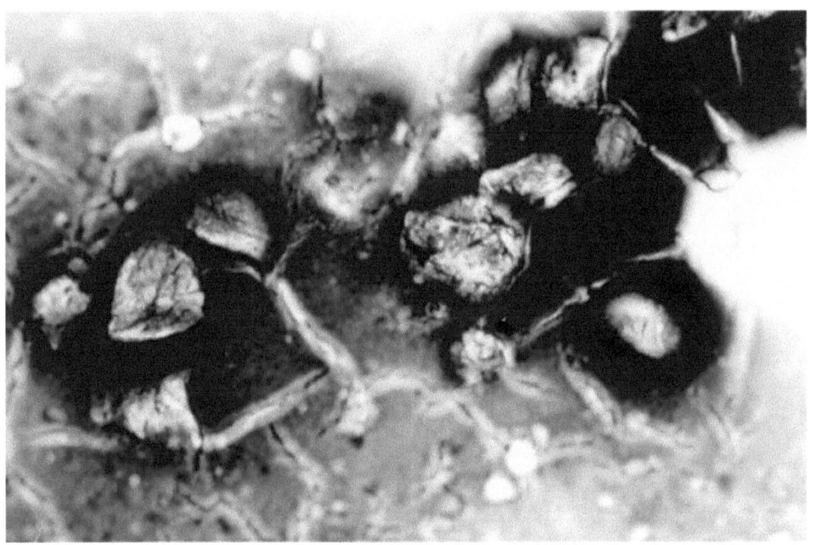

Figure 36 - Calcinosis - CSA - without aspiration. Cancer skin. GIEMSA, 40x.

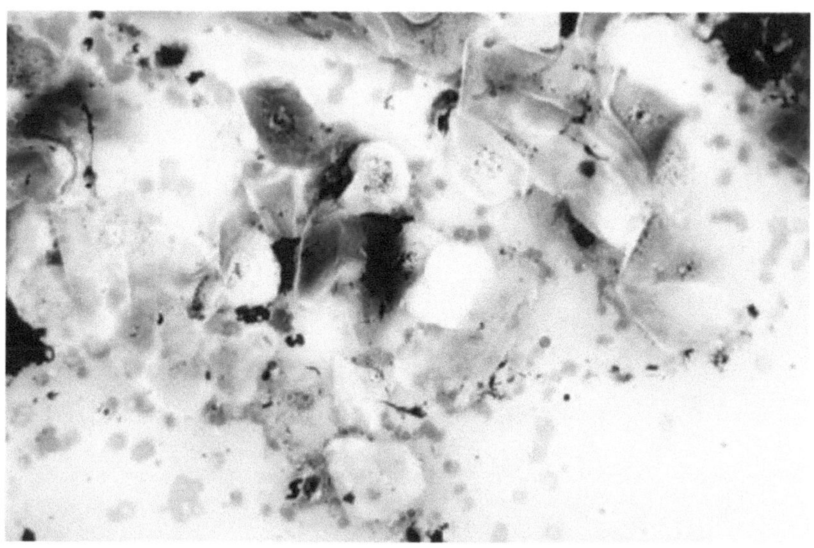

Figure 39 - Epidermoid cyst. CSA - without aspiration. Cancer skin. GIEMSA, 40x.

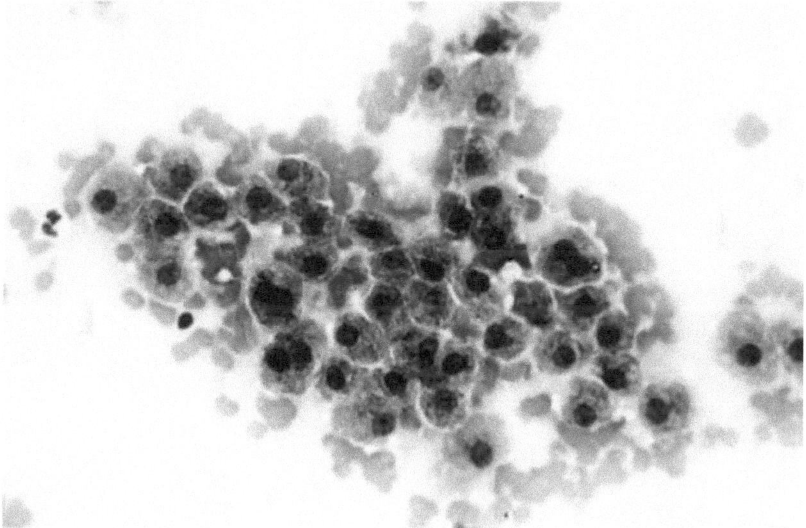

Figura 40 - Hepatic hemosiderosis. CCA - fine needle aspiration. Dog. GIEMSA, 20x.

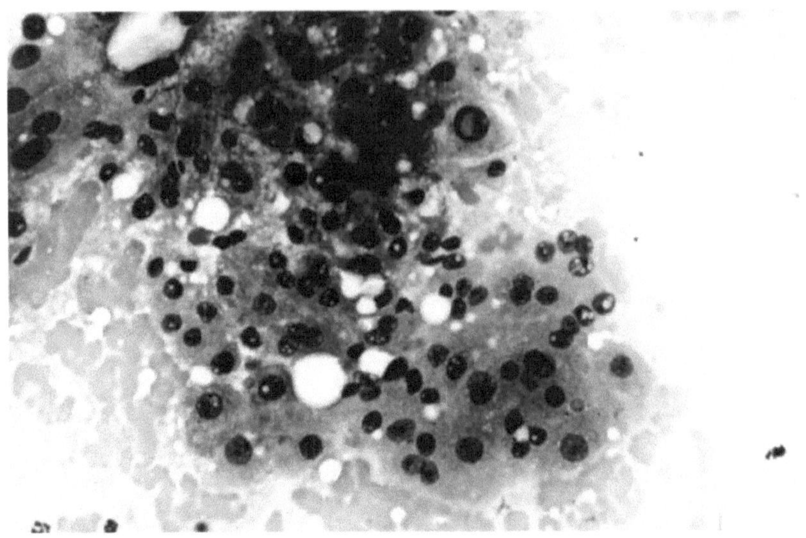

Figura 41 - Hepatic carcinoma. CCA - fine needle aspiration. Dog. GIEMSA, 40x.

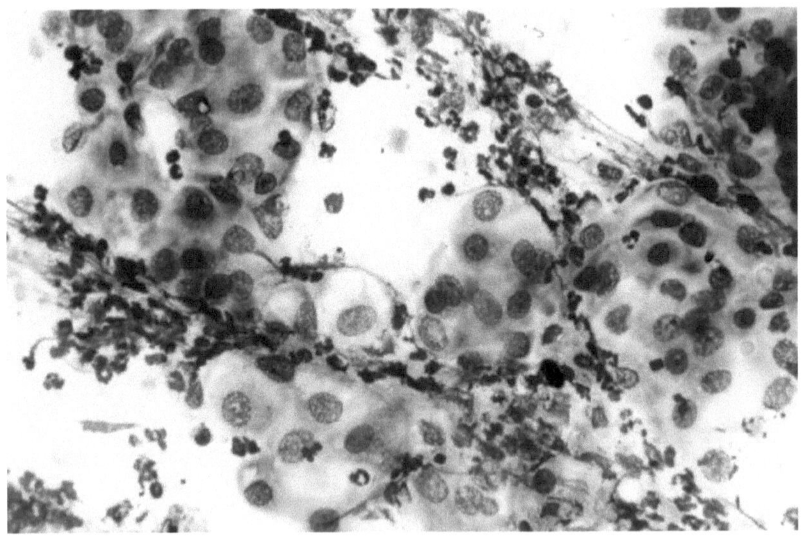

Figure 42 - Carcinoma of the urethra. CEI - cotton swab. Camera. GIEMSA, 40x.

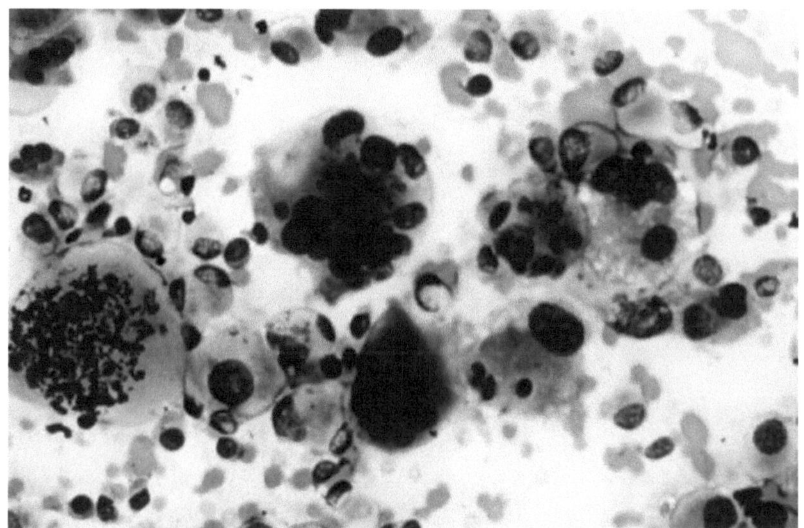

Figure 43 - Breast carcinoma. CCA - fine needle aspiration. Bitch. GIEMSA, 40x.

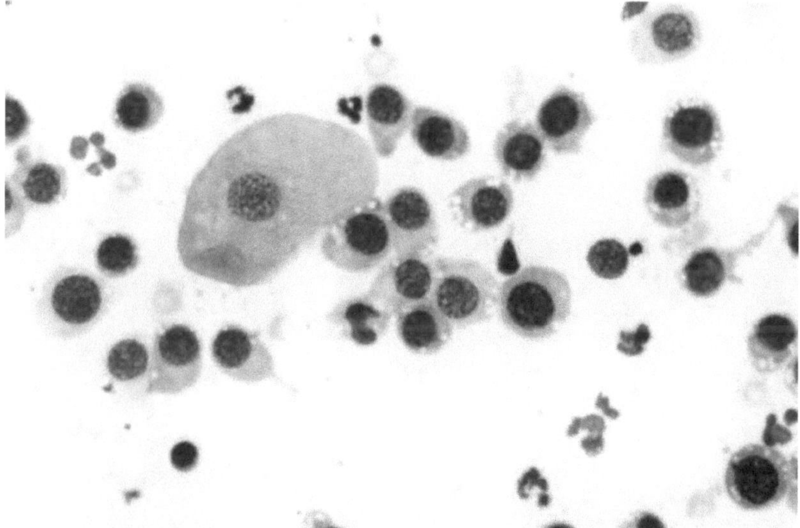

Figura 46 - Cutaneous transmissible venereal tumor - CSA - without aspiration. Cancer skin. GIEMSA, 40x.

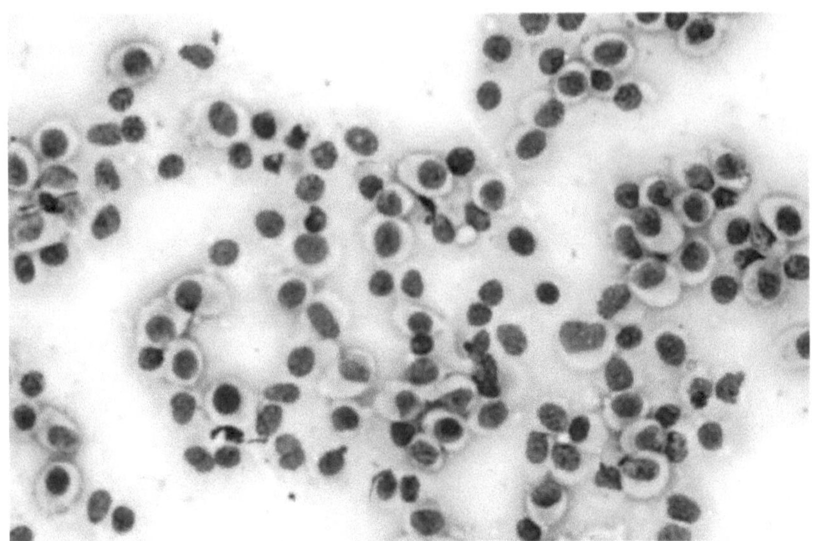

Figura 47 - Cutaneous histiocytoma. CCA - fine needle aspiration. Cancer skin. GIEMSA, 40x.

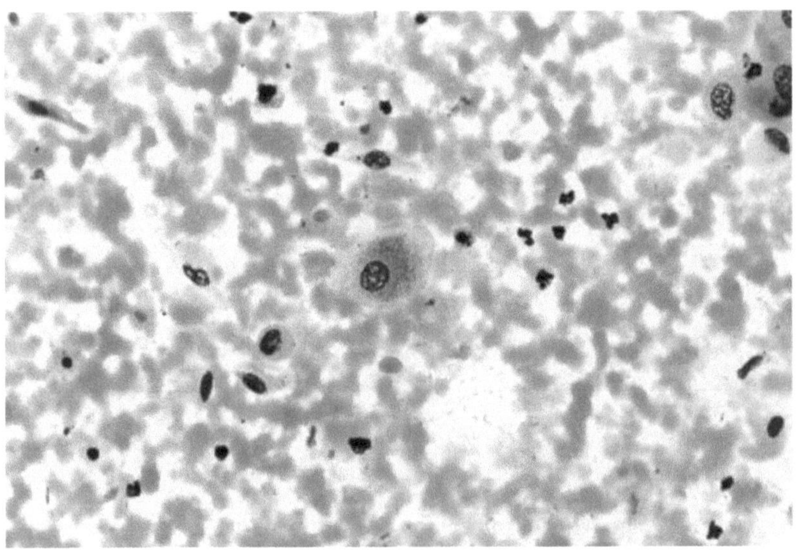

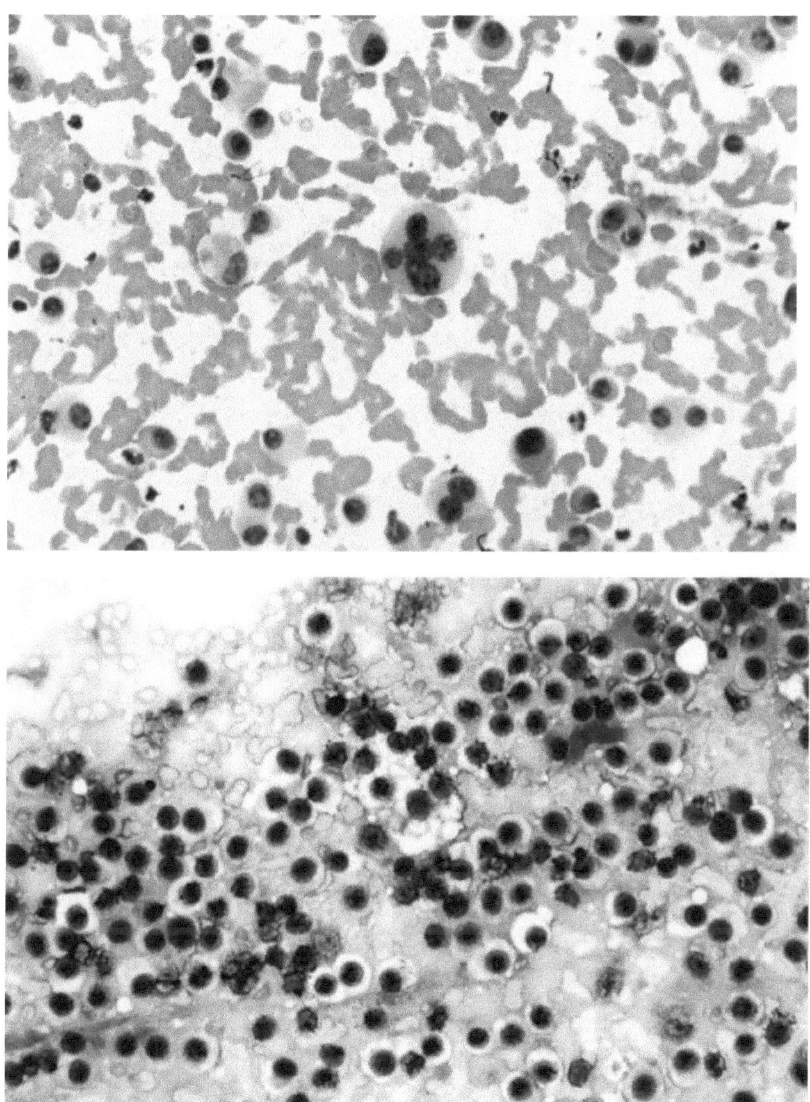

Figura 48 - Mastocytoma under chemotherapy. CSA - no aspiration. Cancer skin. GIEMSA, 40x.

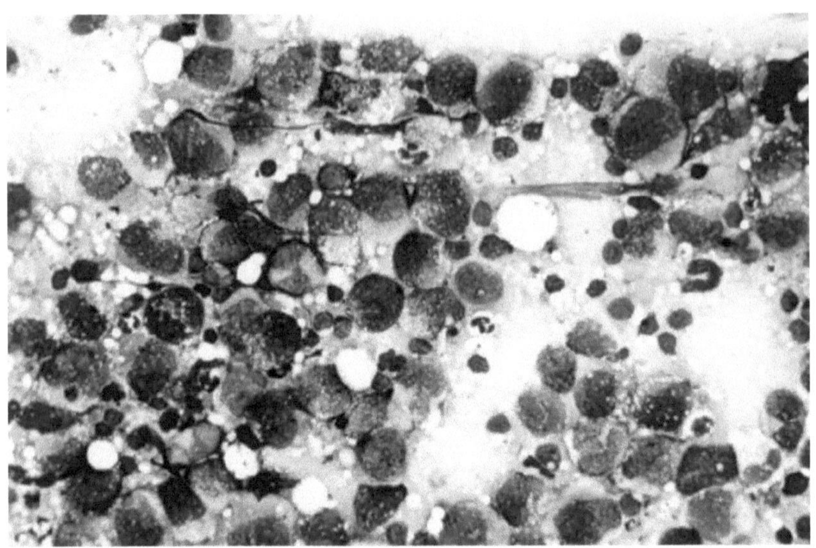

Figura 49 - Cutaneous lymphoma. CCA - fine needle aspiration. Cancer skin. GIEMSA, 40x.

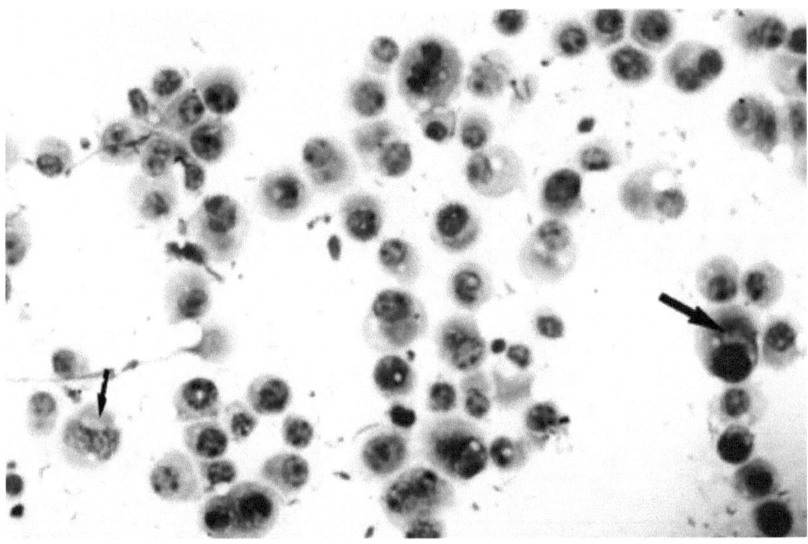

Figura 50 - Cutaneous plasmacytoma. CCA - fine needle aspiration. Golgi complex (arrows). Cancer skin. GIEMSA, 40x.

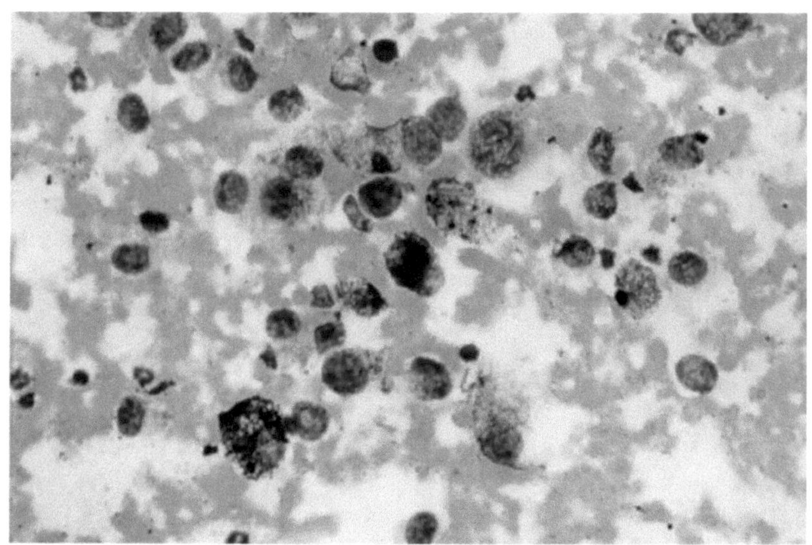

Figura 51 - Cutaneous melanotic melanoma. CCA - fine needle aspiration. Equine skin. GIEMSA, 40x.

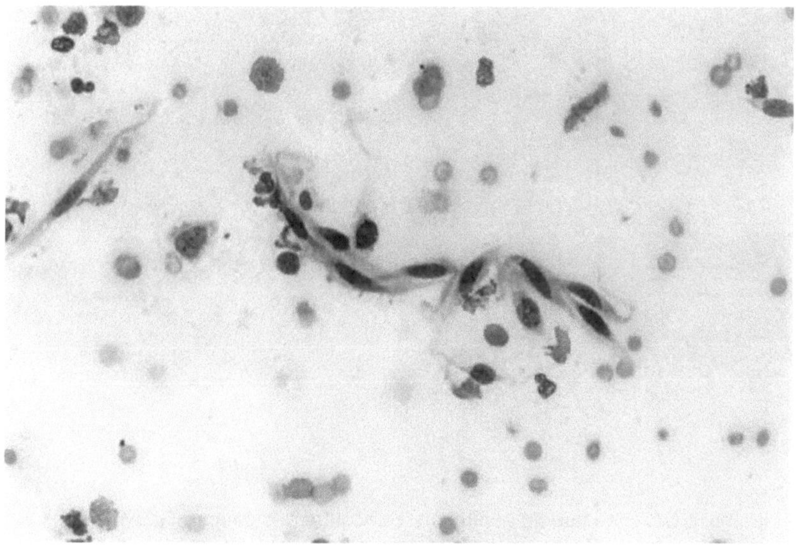

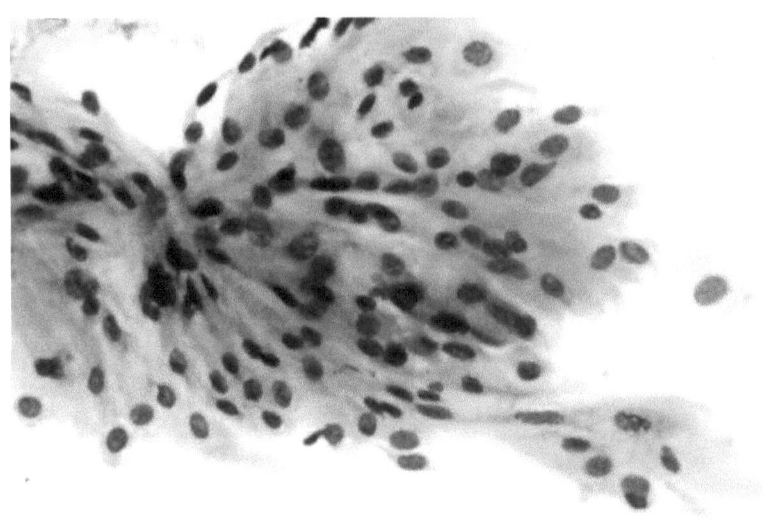

Figure 53 - Synovial sarcoma. Fine needle aspiration. Hip joint. GIEMSA, 40x.

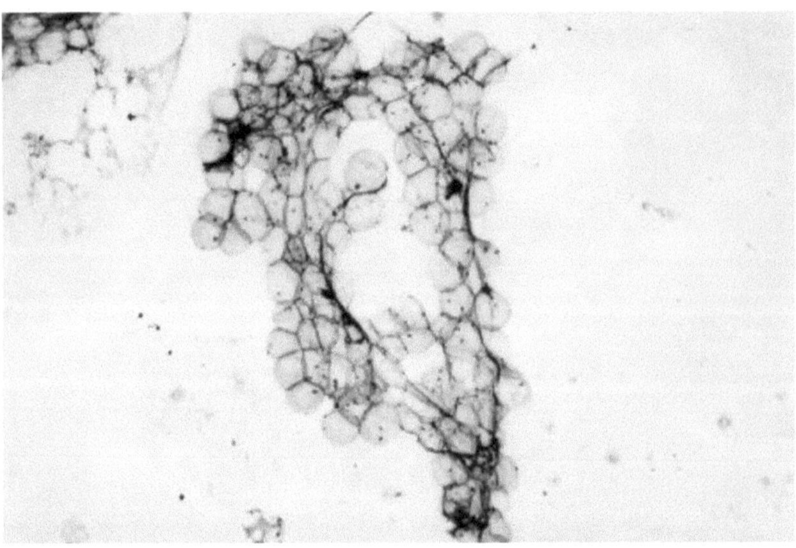

Figura 55 - Lipoma. CCA - fine needle aspiration. Subcutaneous cancer. GIEMSA, 40x.

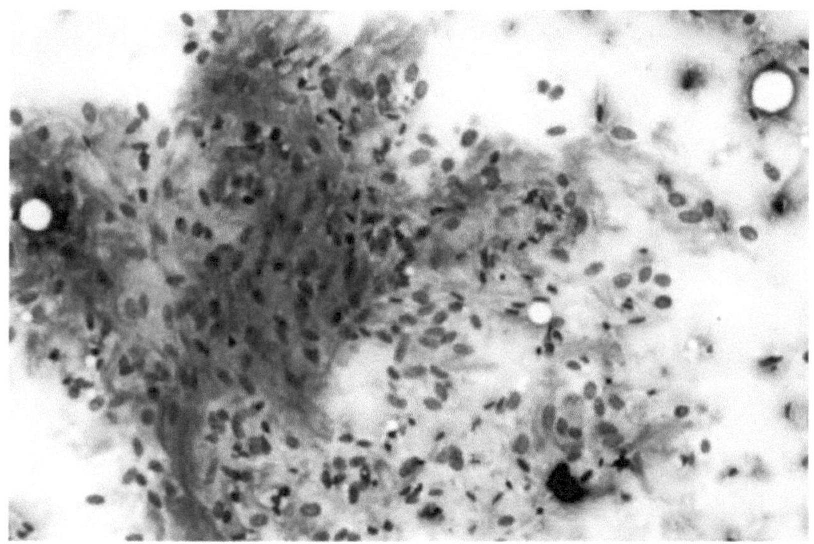

Figura 56 - Complex (mixed) tumor. CCA - fine needle aspiration. Breast of female dog. GIEMSA 40x.

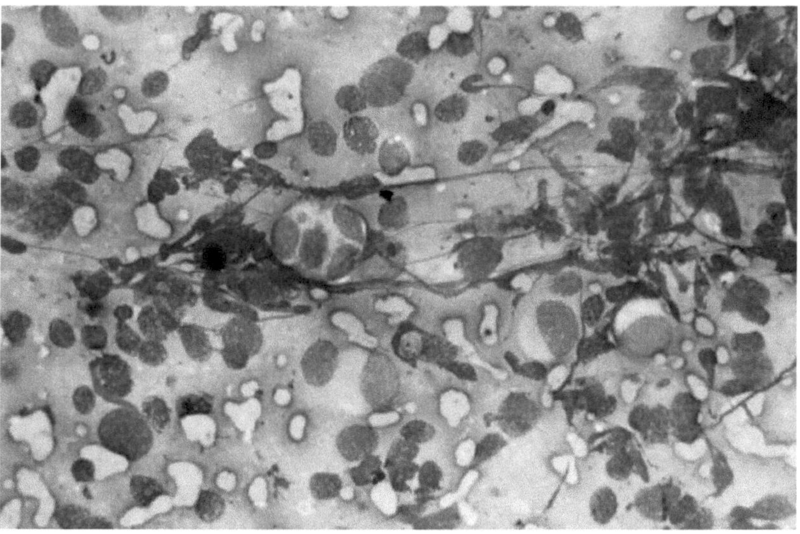

Figure 57 - Seminoma. Fine needle aspiration. Equine. GIEMSA, 40x.

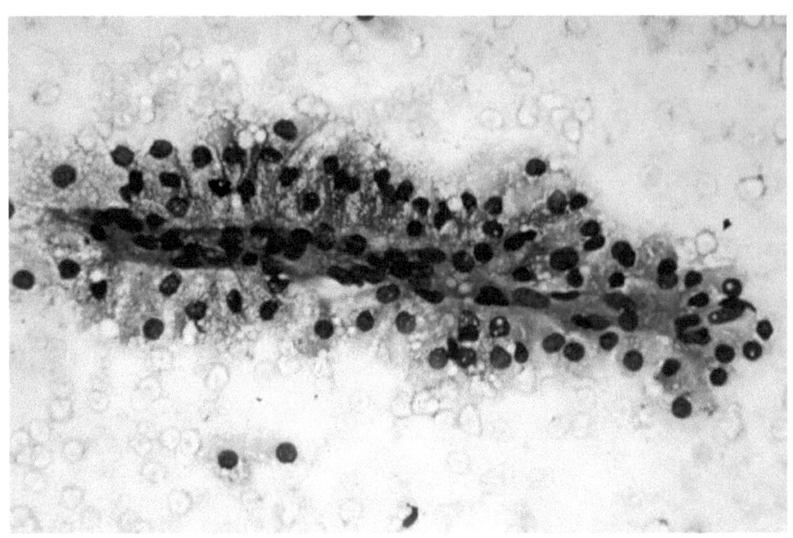

Figure 58 - Interstitial tumor of the testicle. Fine needle aspiration. Dog. GIEMSA, 40x.

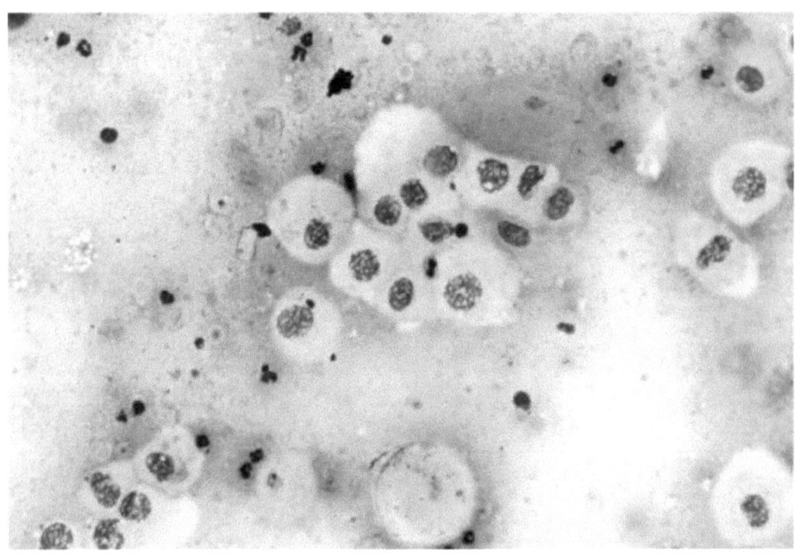

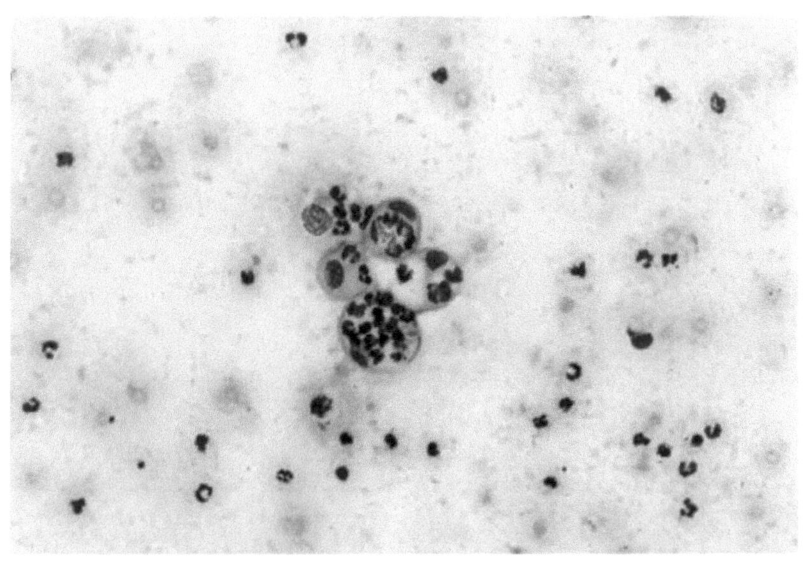

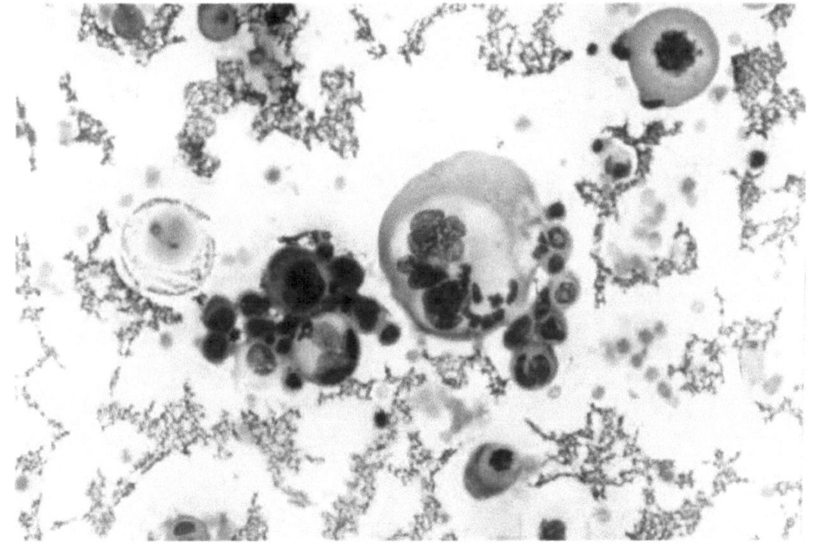

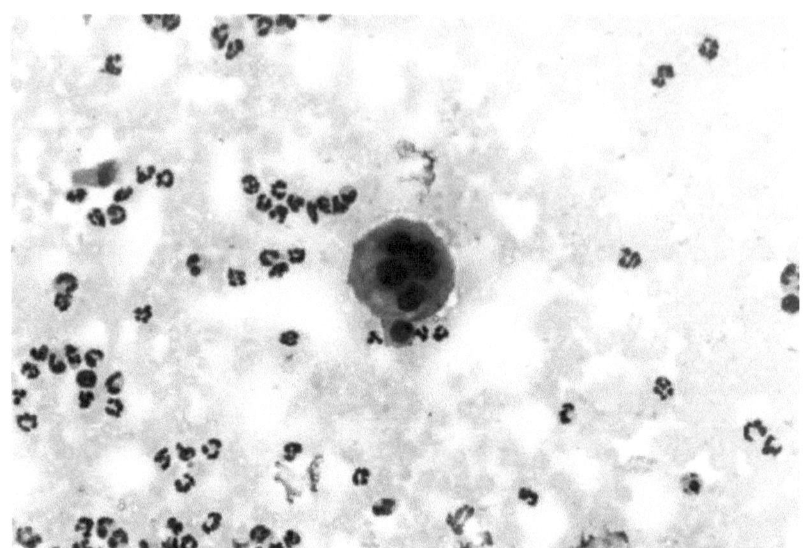

6. Discussion

Even before the use of histological tissue sections on microtomes, professionals used cell morphology to diagnose diseases (KOSS et al., 1984). As early as 1833, Stanly used aspiration cytology to diagnose infectious diseases (STANLY, 1983 apud HAJDU, 1989; TOSTES, 1998). The first reference to the use of cytology in veterinary practice comes from Cole and Evans, in the 1930s, when they included exfoliative cytology as a diagnostic resource (COLE & EVANS apud OBA, 1988).

Around 1850, with the invention of the microtome, the use of paraffin and improvements in staining, histological examination began to be used more frequently than cytological examination (HAJDU, 1989; TOSTES, 1998).

Despite the criticism and resistance that still exists, especially in the veterinary sector in our country, the use of cytological examination has been expanding worldwide, since it offers clinicians speed and safety in diagnosing their patients. Currently, resources such as radiographic images, ultrasound, computerized tomography, electron microscopy analysis, flow cytometry, molecular and enzymology have been incorporated into the examination (KOSS et al. 1984; PERÉZ et al., 1995; MEYER, 1996; MAMPRIN, 1999; WHITE, 2000; ROCHA et al., 2001a; ROCHA et al., 2001b).

The diagnostic accuracy of cytology varies from institution to institution and, before it can be implemented, it is necessary to effectively train professionals with careful quality control (CUNHA, 1987; GUMARÂES et al., 1996; JORNAL, 1997). The aim of this study was to standardize the morphology of inflammatory and non-inflammatory lesions by cytological examination, and to implement and monitor its use in the routine of the Veterinary Hospital at UNESP Botucatu.

Over eight years, 4,953 animals underwent cytological examination using different cell collection techniques. Of these animals, 95.8% had sufficient cytological samples for the diagnosis of inflammatory and non-inflammatory lesions, with only 4.2% of the tests being insufficient, i.e. containing little or no cells for a diagnostic conclusion. The amount of material insufficient for diagnosis is often observed even in the most experienced centers (CUNHA, 1987; GUMARÂES et al., 1996; JORNAL, 1997). The attempt to minimize this problem has been an arduous task that has been achieved step by step, as can be seen by the growing increase in the use of cytology as a diagnostic test over the years.

Insufficient or inconclusive tests should not be ignored from a diagnostic point of view. In these cases, it is important to repeat the examination or use alternative methods to clarify the nature of the lesion (CUNHA, 1987; GUMARÂES et al., 1996; JORNAL, 1997; BOLETIM, 2002). This procedure was always indicated for all animals whose diagnoses were inconclusive. In addition, the absence of cells in the sample associated with the clinical history and imaging gave the work the option of suggesting a diagnosis, as can be explained in the case of mesenchymal tumors, especially those of the bones and vessels. This was the resource used to mitigate the limitations encountered by the techniques.

Several studies have shown that a single technique for collecting cytological samples for diagnostic purposes should not be used, mainly because of the different tissues and locations (COWELL & TYLER, 1989; COWELL et al., 1999; MEYER, 1996; WHITE, 2000). In fact, the use of specific techniques has alleviated the difficulties involved in collecting the material. Thus, the morphological aspects and high cellularity observed in the smears made it possible to diagnose most of the inflammatory and non-inflammatory lesions in the animals submitted to cytological examination during the evaluation period.

For inflammatory lesions, it was observed that not only the presence of inflammatory cells, but their association with cellular modifications including nuclear enlargement, perinuclear halo, hyperchromasia and sometimes binucleation, were essential for the diagnosis of inflammation. These changes, however, are reversible and can be non-specific or associated with an organism and be called specific (MARCONDES, 1975; LAVACH et al., 1977; REPPAS & CANFIELD, 1995; McKEE, 1997; REPPAS & CANFIELD, 2000). These morphological patterns were well characterized in the cytological samples of all species and for both sexes, but with a predominance for the 0 to 5 year age group, which agrees with the numerous reports presented in the literature for both humans and other animals (COWELL & TYLER, 1989; GROSS et al., 1992; KURMAN & SOLOMON, 1994; McKEE, 1997; COWELL et al., 1999; WHITE, 2000).

Cytological examination for the presumptive diagnosis of certain infectious diseases has also been used for scientific research (REPPAS & CANFIELD; 1995; THOMPSON et al., 1997; COWELL & TYLER, 1989;

KURMAN & SOLOMON, 1994; COWELL et al., 1999; DOMINGUES et al., 1999; FARIAS, 2000; RIBEIRO et al., 2002). In the present study, it was possible to report several diagnoses of this nature, such as cryptococcosis, leishmaniasis, filariasis, sporotrichosis, among others.

Cytological samples of non-inflammatory lesions include degenerative, hyperplastic, dysplastic and neoplastic changes. The latter has its own nuclear and cytoplasmic criteria which are sometimes difficult to distinguish from other damaging processes affecting the tissues, but are fundamental for concluding a neoplastic diagnosis (MARCONDES, 1975; BIBBO, 1991; CARVALHO, 1993; REPPAS & CANFIELD, 1995; McKEE, 1997; KOJIMA et al., 1998; MEYER, 1999; WHITE, 2000; SOUZA et al., 2001). In the present study, it was possible to identify all the morphological criteria recommended by these authors and thus identify and classify neoplasms in terms of cell origin and degree of aggressiveness. Epithelial, mesenchymal, round cell and mixed cell origin neoplasms were described. Sequentially, these neoplasms were: carcinomas, osteosarcomas, transmissible venereal tumor, lymphoma, mastocytoma and complex. In this sense, it can be said that the data do not differ from those found in the specific literature (KOSS, 1972; ZACH, 1972; MARCONDES, 1975; COWELL & TYLER, 1989; MOULTON, 1990; MEYER, 1996; DeNICOLA & REAGAN, 1998; MEYER, 1999; ZUCCARI, 1999).

The cases of these processes were significant in animals aged between 6 and 10 years, with a predominance in dogs, especially females. In fact, as has been reported, cancer is the most prevalent disease in dogs in this age group for various reasons, such as more sophisticated methods of diagnosis and lifestyle (MEYER, 1999). The fact that cancer is a chronic process clearly explains the high incidence of this entity in older animals.

During this evaluation there were other important contributions, such as the identification of the morphology of lesions not previously recorded in veterinary scientific literature, neither cytologically nor histologically, such as inflammatory pseudotumor, lactating bladder adenoma, phylloid tumor. In addition to those rarely described such as inflammatory carcinoma and cholestoma; all found in dogs. These cases were sent for consultation to specialized diagnostic centers for men, where there was experience in the subject.

Finally, cytology is an extremely important diagnostic tool for diagnosing inflammatory and non-inflammatory lesions in animals.

7. Conclusion

With the data collected from 1994 to 2002, the following conclusions can be drawn that:

- The cytological examination was efficient in all aspects, except for cases that fell within the limitations of the method, such as mesenchymal neoplasms and those of the central nervous system;
- The cell population of the smears made it possible to morphologically identify lesions not yet recorded in veterinary cytopathology;
- The more experience gained during the course of the work, the better the cytology material was obtained and the better the diagnosis;
- Cell smears from organs with lesions provide sufficient elements to identify and diagnose them, as they stand out from the cell population specific to each organ;
- Cytological examination is an important method for diagnostic investigation.

8. Summary

ROCHA, NS. Cytodiagnosis at the UNESP Botucatu Veterinary Hospital - standardization, implementation and monitoring. Botucatu, 2002, p.94. Thesis (Livre Docência, Disciplina de Anatomia Patològica Geral Veterinària, Departamento de Clinica Veterinària) - Faculdade de Medicina Veterinària e Zootecnia - UNESP - Campus de Botucatu, Universidade Estadual Paulista " Jùlio de Mesquita Filho".

Cytological examination is a method of diagnostic investigation based on cell morphology. Its use is practically unlimited, and it can be used in all superficial lesions or even intracavitary lesions, with the aid of imaging. It is indicated in the control of the therapeutic response, operative procedure, as well as in the investigation of recurrent diseases. The advantages of this test are widely demonstrated in the literature. It is a low-cost procedure, because the material used is simple, and it can be used on an outpatient basis, thus eliminating the need for the patient to be hospitalized. The cytological examination can be carried out on several different sites at the same time, in those animals that may have several lesions. The morphological findings can be used to predict the biological behavior of the lesions, in an attempt to assess prognosis. However, cytological examination is hardly the method of choice for investigating animal diseases in veterinary medical centers. The main aim of this work was to standardize, implement and manage cytological examination in the routine of the Veterinary Pathology Service of the Faculty of Veterinary Medicine and Zootechny at UNESP Botucatu.

For this purpose, from March 23, 1994 to July 11, 2002, in the routine of the Veterinary Hospital, cytological samples were taken by the exfoliative and puncture techniques from all animals that presented cutaneous, subcutaneous, apparent mucosal and intracavitary lesions. Taking into account the species, sex, age group and topography of the lesion, four groups were formed: Group 1, cutaneous and subcutaneous; Group 2, apparent mucous membranes; Group 3, intracavitary and Group 4, lavage.

A total of 4,953 animals with inflammatory and non-inflammatory lesions diagnosed by cytological examination were evaluated, approximately 5.27% of all patients seen at the hospital during this period. The most common method of collection was puncture with aspiration. The most common species was canine. The

1 led the way in the topography of the lesions; animals in all groups aged 0-5 years had the highest number of inflammatory lesions. On the other hand, those in the 6-10 age group led

the way in terms of non-inflammatory processes.

In none of the groups was there any risk to the patient as a result of the material being collected. Analyzing the data on the accuracy of the test, we found that it was possible to diagnose inflammatory and non-inflammatory processes in 95.8% of the tests requested by the Veterinary Hospital. Overall, the results suggest that cytology is an important method in diagnostic research.

Keywords: inflammatory lesion, non-inflammatory, skin, apparent mucosa, fine needle aspiration cytology, capillary cytology, alternative examination, animals.

9. Summary

ROCHA, NS. Cytodiagnostic at Veterinary Hospital at Unesp de Botucatu - to standardize, to implant and to monitor. Botucatu, 2002, p.94. Thesis (Livre Docência), Department of Veterinary Medicine. Discipline of General Veterinary Pathological Anatomy - Faculty of Veterinary Medicine and Zootechny - UNESP - Botucatu Campus, Universidade Estadual Paulista "Jùlio de Mesquita Filho".

The cytologic examination is a method of diagnostic investigation based on cellular morphology. The use is practically unlimited, it can be used in all the superficial lesions or internal organs with image support. There is an indication in the control of the therapeutic answer, operative act, as well as in the research of recidiving disease. The advantages of this examination are widely demonstrated in literature. It's a procedure of low cost, by virtue of utilized material being simple and cheap and, makes possible the use of ambulatory in releasing the patient. There is a possibility of execution in different multiple places, at the same time in those animals that eventually show various lesions. The morphologic characteristics can be used in the identification of biologic behaviors of the lesions, in the attempt of prognostic evaluation. However, the cytologic examination difficultly constitutes in method of choice in investigation of animals illness in the Centers of Veterinary Medicine, especially in our field. The main purpose of this research was to standardize, to implant, and to monitor the cytologic examination in the practice of Pathology service of Faculty of Veterinary Medicine and Zootechny at UNESP Botucatu. From March 23rd , 1994 to July 11th , 2002, in the Veterinary Hospital Practice were collected cytologic samples by exfoliative techniques and punctures of all animals that show cutaneous lesions, subcutaneous, apparent mucous and internal organs. Considering the species, the sex, age distribution, and topography of the lesion were constituted in four groups: G1 - cutaneous and subcutaneous, G2 - apparent mucous, G3 - internal organs and G4 - body fluids. Until the end of this evaluation, 4953 animals porter of inflammatory lesions and no inflammatory diagnosed by cytologic examination participated, approximately 5.27% of all the assistance of the Hospital, in that period. The route of collection most commonly used was the puncture with aspiration. The species, sex and age distribution of the important was canine. The group 1 led in the topography of the lesions. The animals of all groups with a range of 0 to 5 years showed the greatest number of inflammatory lesions. On the other hand, the ones with a range of_6 to 10 years led the non- inflammatory methods. In any group, intercurrences were observed in relation to the patient's risk as a result of the material collection. Analyzing the data referring to the accuracy of the examination, it was observed that it was possible to diagnose inflammatory methods and non-inflammatory in 95.8% of the examinations requested by the Veterinary Hospital. In general, the results allow us to conclude that the cytologic examination is an efficient method in the diagnostic investigation.

Key words: Inflammatory lesions; Non-inflammatory lesions; Skin; Mucous; Cavity; Fine needle aspiration; Fine needle capillary; Alternative examination; Animals.

10. Bibliographical references*

* **NBR 6023**: informaçâo e documentaçâo -Referências - Elaboraçâo, Rio de Janeiro, 2000. 22p.

BIOSIS. Serial sources for the BIOSIS preview database. Philadelphia, 1996. 468p.

ACTA cytologica: The Journal of Clinical Cytology and Cytopathology. St Louis: The International Academy of Cytology, v.42, n.1, jan./feb., 1998. 282p.

ALVES, A. **Urinary cytopathology and evaluation of DNA lesions in dogs with and without clinical manifestations of lower urinary tract disease.** 2001, 119p. Dissertation (Master's Degree) - Faculty of Veterinary Medicine and Zootechny, Universidade Estadual Paulista, Botucatu.

ALBERTS, B.; BRAY, D.; LEWIS, J. et al. **Molecular biology of the cell.** 3.ed. Porto Alegre: Artes Médicas, 1997. 1294p.

AZÙA, J. **Diagnòstico citológico en patologia mamaria.** Barcelona: Espaxs, 1976. 110p.

BAKER, R.; LUMSDEN, J.H. **Color atlas of cytology of the dog and cat.** St. Louis: Mosby, 2000.288p.

BIBBO, M. **Comprehensive cytopathology.** Philadelphia: W.B. Saunders, 1991. 1101p.

BOLETIM SBC. Rio de Janeiro: Brazilian Society of Cytopathology, n.58, jan./feb./mar. 2002. 8p.

BRIDGE, J.A.; ORNDAL, C. Cytogenetic analysis of bone and joint neoplasms. In: HELLIWELL, T.R. (Eds). **Pathology of bone and joint neoplasms.** Philadelphia: W.B. Saunders, 1999. p.59-78.

CARVALHO, G. **Oncological cytology.** Sao Paulo: Atheneu, 1993. 290p.

CORDEIRO, J.L.F.; NEVES, J.P.; FAN, L.C.R. et al. Cervical-uterine cytology for the diagnosis of genital catarrh in cows. **Revista Brasileira de Reproduçâo Animal,** Belo Horizonte, v.13, n.1, p.53-68, 1989.

COWELL, R.L.; TYLER, R.D. Cytology of cutaneous lesions. **Veterinary Clinics of North America: Small Animal Practice**, Philadelphia, v.19, n.4, p.769-794, jul. 1989.

COWELL, R.L.; TYLER, R.D. **Diagnostic cytology and hematology of the horse.** 2.ed. St. Louis: Mosby, 2002. 260p.

COWELL, R.L.; TYLER, R.D.; MEINKOTH, J.H. **Diagnostic cytology and hematology of the dog and cat.** 2.ed. St. Louis: Mosby, 1999. 338p.

CUNHA, M.M.P.L. **Manual de laboratòrio cito-histopatológico.** Brasilia: Ministry of Health Documentation Center, 1987. 44p.

CURTIS, C.F. Diagnostic Techniques and sample collection. **Clinical Techniques in Small Animal Practice,** Philadelphia, v.16, n.4, p.199-206, nov. 2001.

DeMAY, R.M. Fluids In: DeMAY, R.M. (Ed.) **The art & science of cytopathology:** exfoliative cytology. Chicago: American Society of Clinical Pathologists, 1995. p.293294.

DeNICOLA, D.; REAGAN, W.J. Using cytology in the diagnosis of cancer. In: MORRISON, W.B. (Ed.) **Cancer in dogs and cats.** Baltimore: Williams & Wilkins, 1998. p.71-78.

DOMINGUES, P.F. **Study of parameters of milk and blood plasma constituents, possible association of genetic-biochemical polymorphism of beta-lactoglobulins and transferrins and cytological examination in subclinical bovine mastitis.** 1999, 121p. Thesis (PhD) - Faculty of Veterinary Medicine and Zootechny, Universidade Estadual Paulista, Botucatu.

DOMINGUES, P.F.; LANGONI, H.; ROCHA, N.S. et al Fine needle aspiration cytology (FNAC) in mammary glands of cows with subclinical mastitis. **Napgama,** Sao Paulo, v.2, n.4, p.17-19, 1999.

DONAT, E.E.; WOOD, J.; TAO, L. The application of fine needle aspiration cytology in the diagnosis of multiple primary malignant tumors. **Acta Cytologica,** Chicago, v.6, n.33, p.800-804, nov./dez. 1989.

DUCATMAN, B.S.; HOGAN, C.L.; WANG, H.H. A triage system for processing fine needle aspiration cytology specimens. **Acta Cytologica,** Chicago, v.6, n.33, p.797799, nov./dez., 1989.

EMMEL, V.M.; COWDRY, E.V. Collection of specimens, preparation and fixation of smears. In: EMMEL, V.M.; COWDRY, E.V. (Eds). **Laboratory technique in biology and medicine.** Baltimore: Williams & Wilkins, 1964. p.141-152.

EXFOLIATIVE cytology. New York: The American Cancer Society, 1961. 77p.

FRABLE, W.J. Needle aspiration biopsy: past, present and future. **Human Pathology**, Philadelphia, v.20, n.6, p.504-516, jun. 1989.

FARAH, S.B. **DNA: secrets and mysteries.** Sao Paulo: Sarvier, 1997. 276p.

FARIAS, M.R. **Serial clinical, cytopathological and histopathological evaluation of sporotrichosis in cats (*Felis cati* - Linnaeus, 1758) experimentally infected with *Sporothrix schenckii*.** 2000, 97p. Dissertation (Master's Degree) - Faculty of Veterinary Medicine and Zootechny, Universidade Estadual Paulista, Botucatu.

GUIMARAES, E.M.; FERNANDES, P.C.; CERVILHA, N. et al. Fine needle puncture of the breast: results and difficulties. **Jornal Brasileiro de Patologia**, Rio de Janeiro, v.32, n.4, p.153-160,Oct./Nov./Dec. 1996.

GREENE, C.E. **Infectious diseases of the dog and cat.** Philadelphia: W.B. Saunders, 1990. 971p.

GROSS, T.L.; IHRKE, P.J.; WALDER, E.J. **Veterinary dermathopathology: a macroscopic and microscopic evaluation of canine and feline skin disease.** St. Louis: Mosby, 1992. 520p.

HAJDU, S.I. The value and limitations of aspiration cytology in the diagnosis of primary tumors: a symposium. **Acta Cytologica,** Chicago, v.33, n.6, p.741-790, nov./dez. 1989.

JORNAL o patologista. Sao Paulo: Sociedade Brasileira de Patologia, n.48, v.16, feb. 1997. 16p.

KABUKÇUOGLU, F.; KABUKÇUOGLU, Y.; KUZGUN, U. et al. Fine needle aspiration of malignant bone lesions. **Acta Cytologica,** Chicago, v.42, n.4, p.875-882, jul./ago. 1998.

KATE, M.S.; KAMAL, M. BOBHATE, S.K. et al. Evaluation of fine needle capillary sampling in superficial and deep-seated lesions: an analysis of 670 cases. **Acta Cytologica,** Chicago, v.42, n.3, mai./jun. 1998.

KEEBLER, C.M.; SOMRAK, T.M. **The manual of cytotechnology.** 7.ed. Chicago: American Society of Clinical Pathologists, 1993. 464p.

KOJIMA, S.; SEKINE, H.; FUKUI, I. et al. Clinical significance of "cannibalism" in urinary cytology of bladder cancer. **Acta Cytologica,** Chicago, v.42, n.6, p.13651369, nov./dez. 1998.

KOSS, L.G. **Diagnostic cytology and its histopathologic bases.** 2.ed. Philadelphia: Lippincott, 1972. 632p.

KOSS, L.G.; WOYKE, S.; OLSZEWSKI, W. **Aspiration biopsy - cytologic interpretation and histologic bases.** New York: Igaku-Shoin, 1984. 502p.

KURMAN, R.J.; SOLOMON, D. **The Bethesda system for reporting cervical/vaginal cytologic diagnoses.** New York: Springer-Verlag, 1994. 81p.

LAVACH, J.D.; THRALL, M.A.; BENJAMIN, M.M. et al. Cytology of normal and inflamed conjunctivas in dogs and cats. **Journal of American Veterinary Medical Association,** Schaumburg, v.170, n.7, p.722-727, Apr. 1977.

LIMA, M.A.; MAEDA, S.A.; MATTOS, M.C. et al. Fine needle puncture without aspiration (cytopuncture): application of a new technique. **Acta Oncològica Brasileira,** Sao Paulo, v.8, n.3, p.102-104, Sep./Dec. 1988.

MACLEOD, A.G. **Cytology.** Michigan: Upjohn, 1981. 113p.

MAIR, S.; DUNBAR, F.; BECKER, P.J. et al. Fine needle cytology - is aspiration suction necessary? A study of 100 masses in various sites. **Acta Cytologica,** Chicago, v.33, n.6, p.809-813, nov./dez. 1989.

MAMPRIM, M.J. **Diffuse liver disease in dogs: comparative ultrasound study with biochemical tests, biopsy and fine needle aspiration cytology.** 1999, 102p. Thesis (PhD) - Faculty of Veterinary Medicine and Zootechny, Universidade Estadual Paulista, Botucatu.

MARCONDES, N. **Atlas of gynecological cytopathology.** Rio de Janeiro: Atheneu, 1975. 228p.

MAXIMOW, A.A.; BLOOM, W. **A textbook of histology.** Philadelphia: W.B. Saunders, 1942. 695p.

MAZETO, G.M.F.S. **Effect of drug treatment on thyroid cytology and cell proliferation in patients with Graves' disease and its correlation with clinical and laboratory parameters.** 2000, 153p. Thesis (PhD) - School of Medicine, Universidade Estadual Paulista, Botucatu.

McKEE, G.T. **Cytopathology.** Sao Paulo: Arts Médicas, 1997. 361p.

MEYER, D.J. Diagnostic cytology in clinical oncology. In: WITHROW, S.J.; MacEWEN (Eds). **Small animal clinical oncology.** 2.ed. Philadelphia: W.B. Saunders, 1996. p.43-51.

MOONEY, E.E.; LAYFIELD, L.J.; DODD, L.G. Fine-needle aspiration of neural lesions. **Diagnostic Cytopathology,** New York, v.20, n.1, p.1-5, 1999.

MOULTON, J.E. **Tumors in domestic animals.** London: University of California Press, 1990. 672p.

MORRISON, W.B. Diagnostic cytology: common techniques for obtaining cytology smears. In: MORRISON, W.B. (Ed.) **Cancer in dogs and cats.** Baltimore: Williams & Wilkins, 1998. p.71-78.

NOLAN, G.R.; HIRST, L.W.; WRIGHT, R.G. et al. Application of impression cytology to the diagnosis of conjunctival neoplasms. **Diagnostic Cytopathology**, New York, v.11, n.3, p.246-248, 1994.

OBA, E. **Histocytophysiological study of the reproductive activity of buffaloes - *Bubalus bubalis.*** 1988, 83p. Thesis (Livre-docência) - Faculty of Veterinary Medicine and Zootechnics, Universidade Estadual Paulista, Botucatu.

PARIDAENS, A.D.A.; McCARTNEY, A.C.E.; CURLING, O.M. et al. Impression cytology of conjunctival melanosis and melanoma. **British Journal of Ophthalmology,** London, v.76, p.198-201, 1992.

PÉREZ, M.G.; LIESA, J.P.; BURILLO, F.L. et al. Usefulness of urinary enzymology in veterinary medicine. **Veterinary International,** Barcelona, v.7, n.1, p. 2-7, 1995.

RIBEIRO, M.G.; AGUIAR, D.M.; PAES, A.C. et al Cutaneous nocardiosis associated with distemper in dogs. Report of ten cases. **Clinica Veterinària,** v.7, n.39, p. 34-42, jul./ago. 2002.

REPPAS, G.; CANFIELD, P. Citologia diagnòstica de lesiones cutàneas en el perro y en el gato. **Veterinary International,** United Kingdom, v.7, n.1, p.8-30, 1995.

REPPAS, G.; CANFIELD, P Diagnostic cytology of skin lesions. In: ETTINGER, S.J.;

FELDMAN, E.C. (Eds). **Textbook of veterinary internal medicine - diseases of the dog and cat.** 5.ed. Philadelphia: W. B. Saunders, 2000. p.26-29.

ROCHA, N.S. Citologia aspirativa por agulhas finas (CAAF) **Caes e Gatos**, Porto Feliz, v.13, n.75, p.14-16, mai./jun. 1998.

ROCHA, N.S.; BURINI, C.H.P.; LIMA, L.S.A. et al. Use of impression cytology in external ocular diseases in man, cattle and horses. **Revista de Educaçao Continuada**, Sao Paulo, v.4, n.1, p.3-7, 2001a.

ROCHA, N.S.; PERES, J.A.; DINIZ, R. Cytological diagnosis of thyroid gland neoplasia in dogs. **Caes e Gatos**, Porto Feliz, v.15, n.89, p.37, mar./abr. 2000.

ROCHA, N.S.; RAHAL, S.C.; SCHIMITT, F. et al. Fine needle aspiration cytology as an aid during surgery. **Caes e Gatos,** Porto Feliz, v.16, n.98, p.22-23, mai./jun. 2001b.

ROGERS, K.; BARTON, C.L.; HABRON, J. Cytology during surgery. **The Compendium: Small Animal,** v.18, n.2, p.153-163, feb. 1996.

SANDESON, T.L.; PUSTAI, W.; SHELLEY, L. et al. Cytologic evaluation of ocular lesions.

Acta Cytologica, Chicago, v.24, n.5, p.391-400, Sept./Oct. 1980.

SAXE, A.; PHILLIPS, E.; ORFANOU, P. et al. Role of sample adequacy in fine needle aspiration biopsy of palpable breast lesions. **The American Journal of Surgery,** New York, v.182, p.369-371, 2001.

SCOTT, D.W.; MILLER, W.H.; GRIFFIN, C.E. Diagnostic methods. In: SCOTT, D.W.;

MILLER, W.H.; GRIFFIN, C.E. (Eds) **Muller & Kirk's small animal dermatology.** 6.ed. Philadelphia: W.B. Saunders, 2001. p.71-206.

SILVERMAN, J.F.; FINLEY, J.L.; O'BRIEN, K.F. et al. Diagnostic accuracy and role of immediate interpretation fine needle aspiration biopsy specimens from various sites. **Acta Cytologica,** Chicago, v.33, n.6, p.791-796, nov./dez. 1989.

SOUZA, M.L.; TORRES, L.F.; ROCHA, N.S. et al. Peritoneal effusion in a dog secondary to visceral mast cell tumor. **Acta Cytologica,** Chicago, v.45, n.1, p.89-92, jan./feb. 2001.

STERN, R.C.; LIU, K.; DODGE, R.K. et al. Significance of lymphoglandular bodies in bone marrow aspiration smears. **Diagnostic Cytopathology,** New York, v.24, n.4, p.240-243, 2001.

THOMPSON, K.S.; DONZELLI, J.; JENSEN, J. et al. Breast and cutaneous mycobacteriosis: diagnosis by fine-needle aspiration biopsy. **Diagnostic Cytopathology,** New York, v.17, n.1, p.45-49, 1997.

TOSTES, R.A. Cytological Diagnosis in Veterinary Medicine. **Cytological Diagnosis,** p.1-8, 1998. Available at: <http://www.nib.unicamp.br/hvvb/caninos/ tostes.htm>. Accessed on: May 3, 2002.

TSENG, S.C.G. Staging of conjunctival squamous metaplasia by impression cytology. **Ophthalmology**, Rochester, v.92, n.6, p.728-733, jun. 1985.

WIED, G.L.; KOSS, L.G.; REAGAN, J.W. **Compendium on diagnostic cytology.** 5.ed. Chicago: Tutorials of Cytology, 1983. 539p.

WHITE, S.D. The skin as a sensor of internal medical disorders. In: ETTINGER, S.J.; FELDMAN, E.C. (Eds). **Textbook of veterinary internal medicine - diseases of the dog and cat.** 5.ed. Philadelphia: W. B. Saunders, 2000. p.26-29.

YOUNG, J.A. Diagnostic problems in fine needle aspiration cytopathology of the salivary glands. **Journal of Clinical Pathology,** London, v.47, p.193-198, 1994.

ZACH, J. **Citologia practica para internistas.** Barcelona: Salvat, 1972. 176p.

ZAJDELA, A.; ZILLHARDT, P.; VOILLEMOT, N. Cytological diagnosis by fine needle sampling without aspiraton**, Cancer**, Philadelphia, v.59, p.1201-1205, mar. 1987.

ZUCCARI, D.A.P.C. **Contribution to the immunohistochemical study of mammary tumors in bitches.** 1999, 121p. Dissertation (Master) - Faculty of Agricultural and Veterinary Sciences, Universidade Estadual Paulista, Jaboticabal.

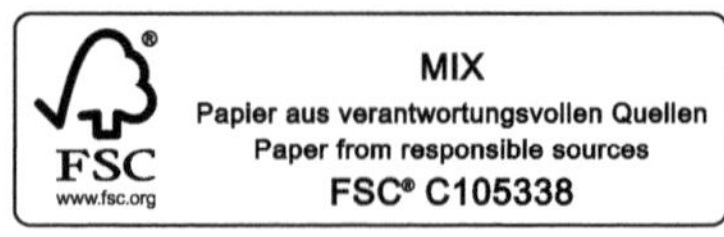

Printed by Books on Demand GmbH, Norderstedt / Germany